AUTHOR'S NOTE

These studies have been published in various journals at different times. They are reprinted together because there is some demand for them, and they are not easily accessible. In preparing them for publication in the present form, some of them have been expanded and all of them have been revised.

While each study is complete in itself, the general thesis running through all of them is the same—that the differences in bodily habit between men and women, particularly the greater strength, restlessness, and motor aptitude of man, and the more stationary condition of woman, have had an important influence on social forms and activities, and on the character and mind of the two sexes.

"Organic Differences in the Sexes" appeared in the *American Journal of Sociology*, III, 31ff., with the title, "On a Difference in the Metabolism of the Sexes;" "Sex and Primitive Social Control," *ibid.*, III, 754ff.; "Sex and Primitive Industry," *ibid.*, IV, 474ff.; "Sex and Primitive Morality," *ibid.*, IV, 774ff.; "The Psychology of Modesty and Clothing," *ibid.*, V, 246ff.; "The Adventitious Character of Woman," *ibid.*, XII, 32ff.; "The Mind of Woman and the Lower Races," *ibid.*, XII, 435ff.; "The Psychology of Exogamy," in the *Zeitschrift für Socialwissenschaft*, V, 1ff., with the title, "Der Ursprung der Exogamie;" "Sex and Social Feeling," in the *Psychological Review*, XI, 61ff., with the title, "The Sexual Element in Sensibility." Portions of a paper printed in the *Forum*, XXXVI, 305ff., with the title, "Is the Human Brain Stationary?" are incorporated in the paper on "The Mind of Woman and the Lower Races," and portions of a paper printed in the *American Journal of Sociology*, IX, 593ff., with the title, "The Psychology of Race-Prejudice," are incorporated in the paper on "Sex and Social Feeling." I acknowledge the courtesy of the editors of these journals for permission to reprint.

W.I.T.

TABLE OF CONTENTS

ORGANIC DIFFERENCES IN THE SEXES

A grand difference between plant and animal life lies in the fact that the plant is concerned chiefly with storing energy, and the animal with consuming it. The plant by a very slow process converts lifeless into living matter, expending little energy and living at a profit. The animal is unable to change lifeless into living matter, but has developed organs of locomotion, ingestion, and digestion which enable it to prey upon the plant world and upon other animal forms; and in contrast with plant life it lives at a loss of energy. Expressed in biological formula, the habit of the plant is predominantly anabolic, that of the animal predominantly katabolic.

Certain biologists, limiting their attention in the main to the lower forms of life, have maintained very plausibly that males are more katabolic than females, and that maleness is the product of influences tending to produce a katabolic habit of body.[1] If this assumption is correct, maleness and femaleness are merely a repetition of the contrast existing between the animal and the plant. The katabolic animal form, through its rapid destruction of energy, has been carried developmentally away from the anabolic plant form; and of the two sexes the male has been carried farther than the female from the plant process. The body of morphological, physiological, ethnological, and demographic data which follows becomes coherent, indeed, only on the assumption that woman stands nearer to the plant process than man, representing the constructive as opposed to the disruptive metabolic tendency.[2]

The researches of Düsing,[3] supplementing the antecedent observations of Ploss,[4] and further supplemented by the ethnological data collected by Westermarck,[5] seem to demonstrate a connection between an abundance of nutrition and females, and between scarcity and males, in relatively higher animal forms and in man. The main facts in support of the theory that such a connection exists are the following: Furriers testify that rich regions yield more furs from females and poor regions more from males. In high altitudes, where nutrition is scant, the birthrate of boys is high as compared with lower altitudes in the same locality. Ploss has pointed out, for instance, that in Saxony from 1847 to 1849 the yield of rye fell, and the birth-rate of boys rose with the approach of high altitudes. More boys are born in the country than in cities, because city diet is richer, especially in meat; Düsing shows that in Prussia the numerical excess of boys is greatest in the country districts, less in the villages, still less in the cities, and least in Berlin.[6] In times of war, famine, and migration more boys are born, and more are born also in poor than in well-to-do families. European statistics show that when food-stuffs are high or scarce the number of marriages diminishes, and in consequence a diminished number of births follows, and a heightened percentage of boys; with the recurrence of prosperity and an increased number of marriages and births, the percentage of female births rises (though it never equals numerically that of the males).[7] More children are born from warm-weather than from cold-weather conceptions,[8] but relatively more boys are born from cold-weather conceptions. Professor Axel Key has shown from statistics of 18,000 Swedish school children that from the end of November and the beginning of December until the end of March or the middle of April, growth in children is feeble. From July-August to November-December their daily increase in weight is three times as great as during the winter months.[9] This is evidence in confirmation of a connection between maleness, slow growth, and either poor nutrition or cold weather, or both. Professor Key's investigations[10] have also confirmed the well-known fact that maturity is reached earlier in girls than in boys and have shown that in respect of growth the ill-nourished girls follow the law of growth of the boys. Growth is a function of nutrition, and puberty is a sign that somatic growth is so far finished that the organism produces a surplus of nutrition to be used in reproduction. Organically reproduction is also a function of nutrition, and, as Spencer pointed out, is to be regarded as discontinuous growth. The fact than an anabolic surplus, preparatory to the katabolic process of reproduction, is stored at an earlier period in the female than in the male, and that this period is retarded in the ill-nourished female, is a confirmation of the view that femaleness is an expression of the tendency to store nutriment, and explains also the infantile somatic characters of woman. Finally, the fact that polyandry is found almost exclusively in poor countries, coupled with the fact that ethnologists uniformly report a scarcity of women in those countries, permits us to attribute polyandry to a scarcity of women and scarcity of women to poor food conditions.

This evidence should be considered in connection with the experiments of Yung on tadpoles, of Siebold on wasps, and of Klebs on the modification of male and female organs in plants:

> According to Yung, tadpoles pass through an hermaphroditic stage, in common, according to other authorities, with most animals.... When the tadpoles were left to themselves, the females were rather in the majority. In three lots the proportion of females to males was: 54-46, 61-39, 56-44. The average number of females was thus about fifty-seven in the hundred. In the first brood, by feeding one set with beef, Yung raised the percentage of females from 54 to 78: in the second, with fish, the percentage rose from 61 to 81; while in the third set, when the especially nutritious flesh of frogs was supplied, the percentage rose from 56 to 92. That is to say, in the last case the result of high feeding was that there were 92 females and 8 males.[11]

> Similarly, the experiments of Siebold on wasps show that the percentage of females increases from spring to August, and then diminishes. We may conclude without scruple that the production of females from fertilized ova increases with the temperature and food supply, and decreases as these diminish.[12]

> Nor are there many facts more significant than the simple and well-known one that within the first eight days of larval life the addition of food will determine the striking and functional differences between worker and queen.[13]

> It is certainly no mere chance, but agrees with other well-known facts, that for the generation of the female organ more favorable external circumstances must prevail, while the male organ may develop under very much more unfavorable conditions.[14]

These facts are not conclusive, but they all point in the same direction, and are probably sufficient to establish a connection between food conditions and the determination of sex. But behind the mere fact that a different attitude toward food determines difference of sex lies the more fundamental —indeed, the real—explanation of the fact, and this chemists and physiologists are not at present able to give us. Researches must be carried farther on the effect of temperature, light, and water on variation, before we may hope to reach a positive conclusion. We can only assume that the chemical constitution of the organism at a given moment conditions the sex of the offspring, and is itself conditioned by various factors—light, heat, water, electricity, etc.—and that food is one of these variables.[15] It is sufficient for our present purpose that sex is a constitutional matter, indirectly dependent upon food conditions; that the female is the result of a surplus of nutrition; and that the relation reported among the lower forms persists in the human species.

In close connection with the foregoing we have the fact, reported by Maupas,[16] that certain Infusorians are capable of reproducing asexually for a number of generations, but that, unless the individuals are sexually fertilized by crossing with unrelated forms of the same species, they finally exhibit all the signs of senile degeneration, ending in death.[17] After sexual conjugation there was an access of vitality, and the asexual reproduction proceeded as before. "The evident result of these long and fatiguing experiments is that among the ciliates the life of the species is decomposed into evolutional cycles, each one having for its point of departure an individual regenerated and rejuvenated by sexual copulation."[18]

The results obtained by Maupas receive striking confirmation in the universal experience of stock-breeders, that, in order to keep a breed in health, it is necessary to cross it occasionally with a distinct but allied variety. It appears, then, that a mixture of blood has a favorable effect on the metabolism of the organism, comparable to that of abundant nutrition, and that innutrition and in-and-in breeding are alike prejudicial.

If this is true, and if heightened nutrition yields an increased proportion of females, we ought to find that breeding-out is favorable to the production of females, and breeding-in to the production of males; and a considerable body of evidence in favor of this assumption exists.[19]

Observations of above 4,000 cases show that, among horses, the more the parent animals differ in color, the more the female foals outnumber the male. Similarly, in-and-in-bred cattle give an excessively large number of bull calves. Liaisons produce an abnormally large proportion of females;[20] incestuous unions, of males.[21] Among the Jews, who frequently marry cousins, the percentage of male births is very high.

> According to Mr. Jacobs' comprehensive manuscript collection of Jewish statistics ... the average proportion of male and female Jewish births registered in various countries is 114.5 males to 100 females, whilst the average proportion among the non-Jewish population of the corresponding countries is 105.25 males to 100 females.... His collection includes details of 118 mixed marriages; of these 28 are sterile, and in the remainder there are 145 female children and 122 male—that is, 118.82 females to 100 males.[22]

The testimony is also tolerably full that among *metis* and among exogamous peoples the female birth-rate is often excessively high.[23]

Viewed with reference to activity, the animal is an advance on the plant, from which it departs by morphological and physiological variations suited to a more energized form of life; and the female may be regarded as the animal norm from which the male departs by further morphological variations. It is now well known that variations are more frequent and marked in males than in females. Among the lower forms, in which activity is more directly determined mechanically by the stimuli of heat, light, and chemical attraction, and where in general the food and light are evenly distributed through the medium in which life exists, and where the limits of variation are consequently small, the constitutional nutritive tendency of the female manifests itself in size. Among many Cephalopoda and Cirripedia, and among certain of the Articulata, the female is larger than the male. Female spiders, bees, wasps, hornets, and butterflies are larger than the males, and the difference is noticeable even in the larval stage. So considerable is the difference in size between the male and female cocoons of the silk-moth that in France they are separated by a particular mode of weighing.[24] The same superiority of the female is found among fishes and reptiles; and this relation, wherever it occurs, may be associated with a habit of life in which food conditions are simple and stimuli mandatory. As we rise in the scale toward backboned and warm-blooded animals, the males become larger in size; and this reversal of relation, like the development of offensive and defensive weapons, is due to the superior variational tendency of the male, resulting in characters which persist in the species wherever they prove of life-saving advantage.[25]

The superior activity and variability of the male among lower forms has been pointed out in great detail by Darwin and confirmed by others.

> Throughout the animal kingdom, when the sexes differ in external appearance, it is, with rare exceptions, the male which has been more modified; for, generally, the female retains a closer resemblance to the young of her own species, and to other adult members of the same group. The cause of this seems to lie in the males of almost all animals having stronger passions than the females.[26]

Darwin explains the greater variability of the males—as shown in more brilliant colors, ornamental feathers, scent-pouches, the power of music, spurs, larger canines and claws, horns, antlers, tusks, dewlaps, manes, crests, beards, etc.—as due to the operation of sexual selection, meaning by this "the advantage which certain individuals have over others of the same sex and species solely in respect of reproduction,"[27] the female choosing to pair with the more attractive male, or the stronger male prevailing in a contest for the female. Wallace[28] advanced the opposite view, that the female owes her soberness to the fact that only inconspicuous females have in the struggle for existence escaped destruction during the breeding season. There are fatal objections to both these theories; and, taking his cue from Tylor,[29] Wallace himself, in a later work, suggested what is probably the true explanation, namely, that the superior variability of the male is constitutional, and due to general laws of growth and development. "If ornament," he says, "is the natural product and direct outcome of superabundant health and vigor, then no other mode of selection is needed to account for the presence of such ornament."[30] That a tendency to spend energy more rapidly should result in more striking morphological variation is to be expected; or, put otherwise, the fact of a greater variational tendency in the male is the outcome of a constitutional inclination to destructive metabolism. It is a general law in the courtship of the sexes that the male seeks the female. The secondary sexual characters of the male are developed with puberty, and in some cases these sexual distinctions come and go with the breeding season. What we know as physiological energy is the result of the dissociation of atoms in the organism; expressions of energy are the accompaniment of the katabolic or breaking-up process, and the brighter color of the male, especially at the breeding season, results from the fact that the waste products of the katabolism are deposited as pigments.

When we compare the sexes of mankind morphologically, we find a greater tendency to variation in man:[31]

All the secondary sexual characters of man are highly variable, even within the limits of the same race; and they differ much in the several races.... Numerous measurements carefully made of the stature, the circumference of the neck and chest, the length of the backbone and of the arms, in various races ... nearly all show that the males differ much more from one another than do the females. This fact indicates that, as far as these characters are concerned, it is the male which has been chiefly modified, since the several races diverged from their common stock.[32]

Morphologically the development of man is more accentuated than that of woman. Anthropologists, indeed, regard woman as intermediate in development between the child and the man.

> The outlines of the adult female cranium are intermediate between those of the child and the adult man; they are softer, more graceful and delicate, and the apophyses and ridges for the attachment of muscles are less pronounced,... the forehead is ... more perpendicular, to such a degree that in a group of skulls those of the two sexes have been mistaken for different types; the superciliary ridges and the glabella are less developed, often not at all; the crown is higher and more horizontal; the brain weight and cranial capacity are less; the mastoid apophyses, the inion, the styloid apophyses, and the condyles of the occipital are of less volume, the zygomatic and alveolar arches are more regular.[33]

Wagner decided that the brain of a woman, taken as a whole, is uniformly in a more or less embryonic condition. Huschke says that woman is always a growing child, and that her brain departs from the infantile type no more than the other portions of her body.[34] Weisbach[35] pointed out that the limits of variation in the skull of man are greater than in that of woman.

Several observers have recorded the opinion that women of dolichocephalic races are more brachycephalic, and women of brachycephalic races more dolichocephalic, than the men of the same races. If this is true, it is a remarkable confirmation of the conservative tendency of woman. "I have thought for several years that woman was, in a general way, less dolichocephalic in dolichocephalic races, and less brachycephalic in brachycephalic races, and that she had a tendency to approach the typical median form of humanity."[36] The skin of woman is without exception of a lighter shade than that of man, even among the dark races. This cannot be due to less exposure, since the women and men are equally exposed among the uncivilized races, but is due to the same causes as the more brilliant plumage of male birds.

The form of woman is rounder and less variable than that of man, and art has been able to produce a more nearly ideal figure of woman than of man; at the same time, the bones of woman weigh less with reference to body weight than the bones of man, and both these facts indicate less variation and more constitutional passivity in woman. The trunk of woman is slightly longer than that of man,[37] and her abdomen is relatively more prominent, and is so represented in art. In these respects she resembles the child and the lower races, i.e., the less developed forms.[38] Ranke states that the typical adult male form is characterized by a relatively shorter trunk, relatively longer arms, legs, hands, and feet, and relatively to the long upper arms and thighs by still longer forearms and lower legs, and relatively to the whole upper extremity by a still longer lower extremity; while the typical female form approaches the infantile condition in having a relatively longer trunk, shorter arms, legs, hands, and feet; relatively to short upper arms still shorter forearms, and relatively to short thighs still shorter lower legs, and relatively to the whole short upper extremity[39] a still shorter lower extremity—a very striking evidence of the ineptitude of woman for the expenditure of physiological energy through motor action.[40]

The strength of woman, on the other hand, her capacity for motion, and her muscular mechanical aptitude are far inferior to that of man. Tests of strength made on 2,300 students of Yale University[41] and on 1,600 women of Oberlin College[42] show the mean relation of the strength of the sexes, expressed in kilograms:

	Back	Legs	Right Forearm
Men	153.0	186.0	56.0
Women	54.0	76.5	21.4

The average weight of the men was 63.1 kilograms, and of the women 51 kilograms; and, making deduction for this, the strength of the men is still not less than twice as great as that of the women. The anthropometric committee reported to the British Association in 1883 that women are little more than half as strong as men.

The first field day of the Vassar College Athletic Association was held November 9, 1895, and a comparison of the records of some of the events with those of similar events at Yale University in the corresponding year gives us a basis of comparison:[43]

	Yale	Vassar
100-yard dash	10-2/5 sec.	15-1/4 sec.
Running broad jump	23 ft.	11 ft. 5 in.
Running high jump	5 ft. 9 in.	4 ft.
220-yard dash	22-3/5 sec.	36-1/4 sec.

Miss Thompson, whose results were obtained in a psychological laboratory, concludes that in reactions where strength is involved men are clearly superior to women, and this is the only respect in which she finds a marked difference:

Motor ability in most of its forms is better in men than in women. In strength, rapidity of movement, and rate of fatigue they have a very decided advantage. These three forms of superiority are probably all expressions of one and the same fact—the greater muscular strength of men. Men are very slightly superior to women in precision of movement. This fact is probably also connected with their superior muscular force. In the formation of a new co-ordination women are superior. The superiority of men in muscular strength is so well known that it is a universally accepted fact. There has been more or less dispute as to which sex displayed greater manual dexterity. According to the present results, that depends on what is meant by manual dexterity. If it means the ability to make very delicate and minutely controlled movements, then it is slightly better in men. If it means ability to co-ordinate movements rapidly to unforeseen stimuli it is clearly better in women.[44]

We have no other than a utilitarian basis for judging some variations advantageous and others disadvantageous. We can estimate them only with reference to activity and the service or disservice to the individual and society implied in them, and a given variation must receive very different valuations at different historical periods in the development of the race. Departures from the normal are simply nature's way of "trying conclusions." The variations which have proved of life-saving advantage have in the course of time become typical, while the individuals in which unfavorable variations, or defects, have occurred have not survived in the struggle for existence. Morphologically men are the more unstable element of society, and this instability expresses itself in the two extremes of genius and idiocy. Genius in general is correlated with an excessive development in brain-growth, stopping dangerously near the line of hypertrophy and insanity; while microcephaly is a variation in the opposite direction, in which idiocy results from arrested development of the brain, usually through premature closing of the sutures; and both these variations occur more frequently in men than in women. There is also evidence that defects in general are more frequent in men than in women.

A committee reported to the British Association for the Advancement of Science, in 1894,[45] that of some 50,000 children (26,287 boys, and 23,713 girls) seen personally by Dr. Francis Warner (1892-94) 8,941 were found defective in some respect. Of these, 19 per cent. (5,112) were boys, and 16 per cent. (3,829) were girls.

An examination of 1,345 idiots and imbeciles in Scotland by Mitchell showed the following distribution of the sexes:

	Male	Female	Male	Female
Idiots	430	284	or 100	to 66.0
Imbeciles	321	310	or 100	to 96.5

showing that "the excess of males is much greater among idiots than among imbeciles; in other words, that the excess of males is most marked in the graver forms of the disease."[46]

A census of the insane in Prussia in 1880 showed that 9,809 males and 7,827 females were born idiots. Koch's statistics of insanity show that in idiots there is almost always a majority of males, in the insane, a majority of females. But the majority of male idiots is so much greater than the majority of female insane that when idiots and insane are classed together there remains a majority of males.[47] Insanity is, however, more frequently induced by external conditions, and less dependent on imperfect or arrested cerebral development. Mayr has shown from statistics of Bavaria that insanity is infrequent before the sixteenth year; and even before the twentieth year the number of insane is not considerable.[48] In insanity the chances of recovery of the female are greater than those of the male, and mortality is higher among insane men than among insane women. There is practical agreement among pathologists on this point.[49] Campbell points out in detail[50] that the male sex is more liable than the female to gross lesions of the nervous system—a fact which he attributes to the greater variability of the male.

An excess of all other anatomical anomalies, except cleft palate, is reported among males. Manley reports that of 33 cases of harelip treated by him only 6 were females.[51] It appears also that supernumerary digits are more frequent in males. Wilder[52] has recorded 152 cases of individuals with supernumerary digits, of whom 86 were males, 39 females, and 27 of unknown sex. A similar relation, according to Bruce, exists in regard to supernumerary nipples.[53]

Muscular abnormalities, monstrosities, deaf-mutism, clubfoot, and transposition of viscera are also reported as of commoner occurrence in men than in women.[54] Lombroso states that congenital criminals are more frequently male than female.[55] Cunningham noted an eighth (true) rib in 14 of 70 subjects examined. It occurred 7 times in males and 7 times in females, but the number of females examined was twice as large as the number of males.[56] The reports of the registrar-general show that for the years 1884-88, inclusive, the deaths from congenital defects (spina bifida, imperforate anus, cleft palate, harelip, etc.) were, taking the average of the five years, 49.6 per million of the persons living in England for the male sex, and 44.2 for the female.[57]

It has already been noted as a general rule throughout nature that the male seeks the female and physicians generally believe that men are sexually more active than women,[58] though woman's need of reproduction is greater,[59] and celibacy unquestionably impresses the character of women more deeply than that of man. Additional evidence of the greater sexual activity of man is furnished by the overwhelmingly large proportion of the various forms of sexual perversion reported by psychiatrists in the male sex.

Pathological variations do not become fixed in the species, because of their disadvantageous nature, but their excess in the male is, as we have seen in the case of variations which have become fixed, an expression of the more energetic somatic habit of the male.

A very noticeable expression of the anabolism of woman is her tendency to put on fat. "Women, as a class, show a greater tendency to put on fat than men, and the tendency is particularly well marked at puberty, when some girls become phenomenally stout."[60] The distinctive beauty of the female form is due to the storing of adipose tissue, and the form even of very slender women is gracefully rounded in comparison with that of man. Bischoff found the following relation between muscle and fat in a man of 33, a woman of 22, and a boy of 16, all of whom died accidentally and in good physical condition:

	Man	Woman	Boy
Muscle	41.18	35.8	44.2

Fat	18.2	28.2	13.9

The steatopyga of the women of some races and the accumulation of adipose tissue late in life are quasi-pathological expressions of this tendency.

In tracing the transition from lower to higher forms of life, we find a great change in the nature of the blood, or what answers to the blood, and the constitution of the blood is some index of the intensity of the metabolic processes going on within the organism. The sap of plants is thin and watery, corresponding with the preponderant anabolism of the plant. "Blood is a peculiar kind of sap," and there is almost as much difference between this sap in warm-blooded and cold-blooded animals as between the latter and plants. Rich, red blood characterizes the forms of life fitted for activity and bursts of energy. In his exhaustive work on the blood Hayem has given a summary of the results of the investigations of chemists and physiologists on the differences in the composition of the blood in the two sexes. Contrary to the assertion of Robin, Hayem finds that the white blood-corpuscles are not more numerous in women than in men, and he also states that the number of hæmatoblasts is the same in the two sexes. All chemists are agreed, however, that the number of red corpuscles is greater in men than in women. Nasse found in man 0.05824 of iron to 100, and in woman only 0.0499. Becquerel and Rodier give 0.0565 for man, 0.0511 for woman, and Schmidt, Scherer, and others give similar results. Welcker (using a chromometer) found between the corpuscles of man and woman the relation of 5 to 4.7, and Hayem confirmed this by numeration. Cadet found in woman on the average 4.9 million corpuscles per cubic millimeter, and in man 5.2 million. More recently Korniloff, using still another method—the spectroscope of Vierordt—has reached about the same result. The proportion of red blood-corpuscles varies according to individual constitution, race, and sex. In robust men Lacanu found 136 red corpuscles in 1,000; in weak men, only 116 in 1,000; in robust women, only 126 in 1,000; and in weak women, 117.[61] Professor Jones has taken the specific gravity of the blood of above 1,500 individuals of all ages and of both sexes.[62] An examination of his charts shows that the specific gravity of the male is higher than that of the female between the ages of 16 and 68. Between the ages of 16 and 45 the average specific gravity of the male is about 1,058, and that of the female about 1,054.5. At 45 years the specific gravity of the male begins to fall rapidly and that of the female to rise rapidly, and at 55 they are almost equal; but the male remains slightly higher until 68 years, when it falls below that of the female. The period of marked difference in the specific gravity of the blood is thus seen to be coincident with the period of menstruation in the female. A chart constructed by Leichtenstern, based upon observations on 191 individuals and showing variations in the amount of hæmoglobin with age, is also reproduced by Professor Jones, suggesting that the variations in specific gravity of the blood with age and sex are closely related to variations in the amount of hæmoglobin. Leichtenstern states that the excess in men of hæmoglobin is 7 per cent. until the tenth year, 8 per cent. between 11 and 50 years, and 5 per cent. after the fiftieth year.[63] Jones states further[64] that the specific gravity is higher in persons of the upper classes and lower in the poorer classes. Observations of boys who were inmates of workhouses gave a mean specific gravity of 1,052.8 and on schoolboys a mean of 1,056, while among the undergraduate students of Cambridge University he found a mean of 1,059.5. Several men of very high specific gravity in the last group had distinguished themselves in athletics. "Workhouse boys are in most cases of poor physique, and one can hardly find a better antithesis than the general type of physique common among the athletic members of such a university as Cambridge."[65] There is no more conclusive evidence of an organic difference between man and woman than these tests of the blood. They permit us to associate a high specific gravity, red corpuscles, plentiful hæmoglobin, and a katabolic constitution.

A comparison of the waste products of the body and of the quantity of materials consumed in the metabolic process indicates a relatively larger consumption of energy by man. It is stated that man produces more urine than woman in the following proportion: men, 1,000 to 2,000 grams daily; women, 1,000 to 1,400 grams. As age advances, the amount diminishes absolutely and relatively in proportion to the diminution of the energy of the metabolic process. A table prepared from adults of both sexes, twenty-five years of age, of the average weight of sixty kilograms, shows a larger proportion both of inorganic and organic substances in the urine of men.[66] Milne Edwards has found that the bones of the male are slightly richer in inorganic substances than those of the female.[67]

The lung capacity of women is less, and they consume less oxygen and produce less carbonic acid than men of equal weight, although the number of respirations is slightly higher than in man. On this account women suffer deprivation of air more easily than men. They are not so easily suffocated, and are reported to endure charcoal fumes better, and live in high altitudes where men cannot endure the deprivation of oxygen.[68] The number of deaths from chloroform is reckoned as from two to four times as great in males as in females, and this although chloroform is used in childbirth. Children also bear chloroform well.[69] Women, like children, require more sleep normally than men, but "Macfarlane states that they can better bear the loss of sleep, and most physicians will agree with him.... One of the greatest difficulties we have to contend with in nervous men is sleeplessness, a result, no doubt, of excessive katabolism."[70] Loss of sleep is a strain which, like gestation, women are able to meet because of their anabolic surplus. The fact that women undertake changes more reluctantly than men, but adjust themselves to changed fortunes more readily, is due to the same metabolic difference. Man has, in short, become somatically a more specialized animal than woman, and feels more keenly any disturbance of normal conditions, while he has not the same physiological surplus as woman with which to meet the disturbance.

Lower forms of life have the remarkable quality of restoring a lost organ, and of living as separate individuals if divided. This power gradually diminishes as we ascend the scale of life, and is lost by the higher forms. It is a remarkable fact, however, that the lower human races, the lower classes of society, women and children, show something of the same quality in their superior tolerance of surgical disease. The indifference of savage races to wounds and loss of blood has everywhere been remarked by ethnologists. Dr. Bartels has formulated the law of resistance to surgical and traumatic treatment in the following sentence: "The higher the race, the less the tolerance, and the lower the culture-condition in a given race, the greater the tolerance."[71] The greater disvulnerability of women is generally recognized by surgeons. The following figures from Lawrie, Malgaigne, and Fenwick are representative:[72]

LAWRIE(GLASGOW)

	Men	Deaths	Women	Deaths
Pathological amputations	110 cases	29	41 cases	7
Traumatic amputations	106 "	59	14 "	4
Total	216 cases	88	55 cases	11
	or, 40.74 deaths per 100		20 deaths per 100	

A difference of 20.74 per cent. in favor of women.

MALGAIGNE (HOSPITALS OF PARIS)

	Men	Deaths	Women	Deaths
Major pathological amputations	280 cases	138	98 cases	44
Minor pathological amputations	106 cases	9	40 cases	2
Major traumatic amputations	165 "	107	17 "	10
Minor traumatic amputations	73 "	13	10 "	0
Total	624 cases	267	165 cases	56
	or, 37.98 deaths per 100		34.18 deaths per 100	

A difference of 3.8 per cent. in favor of women.

FENWICK (NEWCASTLE, GLASGOW, EDINBURGH)

	Men	Deaths	Women	Deaths
Amputations	304 cases	86	64 cases	16
	or, 27.86 deaths per 100		25 deaths per 100	

A difference of 2.86 per cent. in favor of women.

TOTAL FOR THE THREE SERIES

	Men	Deaths	Women	Deaths
Amputations	1144 cases	441	284 cases	83
	or, 38.56 deaths per 100		29.29 deaths per 100	

A difference of 9.27 per cent. in favor of women.

Legouest states in the same article that the lowest mortality of all is in children from 5 to 15 years of age. Ellis quotes a passage from a paper read by Lombroso at the International Congress of Experimental Psychology held in London:

> Billroth experimented on women when attempting a certain operation (excision of the pylorus) for the first time, judging that they were less sensitive and therefore more *disvulnerable*, i.e., better able to resist pain. Carle assured me that women would let themselves be operated upon almost as though their flesh were an alien thing. Giordano told me that even the pains of childbirth caused relatively little suffering to women, in spite of their apprehensions. Dr. Martini, one of the most distinguished dentists of Turin, has informed me of the amazement he has felt at seeing women endure more easily and courageously than men every kind of dental operation. Mela, too, has found that men will, under such circumstances, faint oftener than women.[73]

The same tolerance of pain and misery in women is shown by an examination of the number of male and female suicides from physical suffering. Von Oettingen states that in 30,000 cases the percentage of suicides from physical suffering was in men 11.4, in women 11.3;[74] and Lombroso, following Morselli, gives the following table representing the proportion out of a hundred suicides of each sex resulting from the same cause:[75]

	Men	Women
Germany (1852-61)	9.61	8.08
Prussia (1869-77)	6.00	7.00
Saxony (1875-78)	4.61	6.21
Belgium	1.34	0.84
France (1873-78)	14.28	13.56
Italy (1866-77)	6.70	8.50
Vienna (1851-59)	9.20	10.04
Vienna (1869-78)	7.73	70.37
Paris (1851-59)	10.27	11.22
Madrid (1884)	31.81	31.25

But these figures represent the numbers of suicides in each hundred of either sex, whereas suicide is three to four times as frequent among men as among women, and the absolute proportion of suicide among men from physical pain is, therefore, overwhelmingly great. Still more significant is a table given by Lombroso showing the percentage of suicides from want:[76]

	Men	Women
Germany (1852-61)	37.75	18.46
Saxony (1875-78)	6.64	1.52
Belgium	4.65	4.02
Italy (1866-77)	7.00	4.60
Italy (1866-77) (financial reverses)	12.80	2.20
Norway (1866-70)	10.30	4.50
Vienna (1851-59)	6.64	3.10

But the excess of male suicides over females is so great that, reckoned absolutely, about one woman to seven or ten men is driven by want to take her life.

Physical suffering and want are among the motives which, constitutional differences aside, would appeal with about the same force to the two sexes. But the great excess both of suicide (3 or 4 men to 1 woman) and of crime (4 or 5 men to 1 woman) in men, while directly conditioned by a manner of life more subject to vicissitude and catastrophe, is still remotely due to the male, katabolic tendency which has historically eventuated in a life of this nature in the male.

Woman offers in general a greater resistance to disease than man. The following table from the registrar-general's report for 1888[77] gives the mortality in England per million inhabitants at all ages and for both sexes from 1854 to 1887 in a group of diseases chiefly affecting young children:

Disease	Year	Male	Female
Smallpox	1854-87	183	148
Measles	1848-87	426	408

Scarlet fever	1859-85	763	738
Diphtheria	1859-87	157	176
Croup	1848-87	221	192
Whooping-cough	1848-87	451	554
Diarrhoea, dysentery	1848-87	932	835
Enteric fever	1869-87	288	277

or, a total mortality of 3,421 per million for the males and 3,328 for the females. The greater fatality of diphtheria and whooping-cough in the female is attributed to the smaller larynx of girls, and to their habit of kissing. In diphtheria, indeed, the number of girls attacked is in excess of that of the boys, and it does not appear that their mortality is higher when this is considered.[78] Statistics based on nearly half a million deaths from scarlet fever in England and Wales (1859-85) show a mean annual in males of 778, and in females of 717, per million living.[79] Dr. Farr reports on the mortality from cholera in the epidemic years of 1849, 1854, and 1866, that

the mean mortality from all causes in the three cholera years was, for males, 19.3 in excess, for females, 17.0 in excess of the average mortality to 10,000 living; so females suffered less than males.... The mortality is higher in boys than in girls at all ages under 15; at the ages of reproduction, 25 to 45, the mortality of women, many of them pregnant, exceeds the mortality of men; but at the ages after 65 the mortality of men exceeds the mortality of women.[80]

Statistics show that woman is more susceptible to many diseases, but in less danger than man when attacked, because of her anabolic surplus, and also that the greatest mortality in woman is during the period of reproduction, when the specific gravity of the blood is low and her anabolic surplus small. It is significant also that the point of highest mortality from disease and of the highest rate of suicide in the female, as compared with the male, falls at about 15 years, and is to be associated with the rapid physiological changes preceding that time.[81]

The numerical relation of the sexes at birth seems to be more variable in those regions where economic conditions and social usages are least settled, but in civilized countries the relation is fairly constant, and statistics of 32 countries and states between the years 1865 and 1883 show that to every 100 girls 105 boys are born, or including stillborn, 100 girls to 106.6 boys.[82] But the mortality of male children so much exceeds that of female that at the age of five the sexes are about in numerical equilibrium; and in the adult population of all European countries the average numerical relation of the sexes is reckoned as 102.1 women to 100 men. Von Oettingen gives a representative table;[83] compiled from statistics of eight European countries, showing that (omitting the stillborn) 124.71 boys to 100 girls die before the end of the first year, and that between the years of 2 and 5 the proportion is 102.91 boys to 100 girls; or, about 25 per cent. excess of boys in the first year, and 3 per cent. in the years between 1 and 5. In the intra-uterine period and at the very threshold of life the mortality of males is still greater. The figures of Wappaeus were 100 stillborn girls to 140.3 boys; Quetelet gave the proportion as 100:133.5; and the statistics of fourteen European countries during the years 1865-83 show that 130.2 boys were stillborn to every 100 girls.[84] So that, while more boys than girls are born living, still more are born dead. That this astonishingly high mortality is due in part to the somewhat larger size of boys at birth and the narrowness of the maternal pelvis is indicated by the statement of Collins, of the Rotunda Lying-in Hospital, Dublin, that within half an hour after birth only 1 female died to 16 males; within the first hour 2 females to 19 males; and within the first 6 hours, 7 females to 29 males.[85] But that this explanation is not sufficient is shown by the fact that a high mortality of boys extends through the whole of the first year, and through five years, in a diminishing ratio, and also that the tenacity of woman on life, as will be shown immediately, is greater at every age than man's except during a period of about five years following puberty. "There must be," says Ploss, "some cause which operates more energetically in the removal of male than of female children just before and after birth;"[86] but, besides the more violent movement of boys and their greater size, no explanation of the cause has been advanced more acceptably than Haushofer's teleological one, quoted by Ploss, that Nature wished to make a more perfect being of man and therefore threw more obstacles in his way. A satisfactory explanation is found if we regard the young female as more anabolic, and more quiescent, with a stored surplus of nutriment by which in the helpless and critical period of change from intra- to extra-uterine conditions it is able to get its adjustment to life. The constructive phase of metabolism has prevailed in them even during fetal life. That there is need of a surplus of nutrition in the child at birth, or that a surplus will stand it in good stead, is indicated by the results of the weighing of children communicated by Winckel to the Gynaecological Society in Berlin in 1862. Winckel weighed 100 new-born children, 56 boys and 44 girls, showing that birth was uniformly followed by a loss of weight. The average diminution was about 108 grams the first day, and but little less the second day. At the end of five days the loss was 220 grams, six-sevenths of which occurred during the first two days.[87] The tendency to decreased vitality in girls after maturity and before marriage, just referred to, must be associated with the katabolic changes implied in menstruation and the newness to the system of this destructive phase of metabolism.

We should expect the death-rate of men to run high during the period of manhood, in consequence of their greater exposure to peril, hardship, and the storm and stress of life. But two tendencies operate to reduce the comparative mortality of men between the twentieth and about the fortieth year: the fact of the severe male mortality in infancy, which has removed the constitutionally weak contingent, and the fact that during this period women are subject to death in connection with childbirth. So that in the prime of life the mortality of males does not markedly exceed that of females. But the statistics of longevity show that with the approach of old age the number of women of a given age surviving is in excess of the men, and that their relative tenacity of life increases with increasing years. Ornstein has shown, from the official statistics of Greece from 1878 to 1883, that in every period of five years between the ages of 85 and 110 years and upward a larger number of women survive than of men, and in the following proportion:

Years	Men	Women
85-90	1,296	1,347
90-95	700	820
95-100	305	370
100-105	116	168
105-110	52	69

110 and over	20	34

Of the 459 centenarians 188 were men and 271 were women.[88] In Bavaria the women aged from 51 to 55 years alive in 1874 had lived in the aggregate more than seven million years, while the men of the same age had lived not so much as six and one-half million.[89] Turquan[90] gives a table showing the death-rate of centenarians in all France during a period of twenty years (1866-85). From this it appears that there died in these years an annual average of 73 centenarians, of whom 27 were men and 46 women. In only one year of the twenty did the deaths of men exceed those of women. Lombroso and Ferrero have shown that between 1870 and 1879 the inhabitants of the prisons and convict establishments in Italy who were over 60 years of age showed a percentage of 4.3 among the women, and 3.2 among the men, although the number of men condemned to prison for long periods is far greater than among women.

> Women are not only longer-lived than men, but have greater powers of resistance to misfortune and deep grief.
>
> This is a well-known law, which in the case of the female criminal seems almost exaggerated, so remarkable is her longevity and the toughness with which she endures the hardships, even the prolonged hardships, of prison life.... I know some denizens of female prisons who have reached the age of 90, having lived within those walls since they were 29 without any grave injury to health.[91]

Woman's resistance to death is thus more marked at the two extremes of life, infancy and old age, the periods in which her anabolism is uninterrupted. Menstruation, reproduction, and lactation are at once the cause of an anabolic surplus and the means of getting rid of it. At the extremes of life no demand of this kind is made on woman, and her anabolic nature expresses itself at these times in greater resistance.

Dr. Lloyd Jones has determined that between 17 and 45 years of age the specific gravity of the blood of women is lower than that of men. In old women the specific gravity rises above that of old men, and he suggests that their greater longevity is due to this.[92] No doubt the greater longevity of women is to be associated with the rise in specific gravity of their blood, but this rise in the specific gravity of women after 45 years is consequent upon their anabolic constitution. High specific gravity in general is associated with abundant and rich nutrition; it falls in women during pregnancy, lactation, and menstruation, and when these functions cease it is natural that the constructive metabolic tendency on which they are dependent should show itself in a heightened specific gravity of the blood (i.e., greater richness), and in consequence greater longevity.

Some facts in the brain development of women point to the same conclusion. The growth of the brain is relatively more rapid in women than in men before the twentieth year. Between 15 and 20 it has reached its maximum, and from that time there is a gradual decline in weight until about the fiftieth year, when there is an acceleration of growth, followed by a renewed diminution after the sixtieth year. The maximum of brain weight is almost reached by men at 20 years, but there is a slow increase until 30 or 35 years. There is then a diminution until the fiftieth year, followed by an acceleration, and at 60 years again a rapid diminution in weight; but the acceleration is more marked and the final diminution less marked in woman than in man.[93] A table prepared by Topinard shows that woman from 20 to 60 years of age has from 126 to 164 grams less brain weight than man, while her deficit from 60 to 90 years is from 123 to 158 grams.[94]

The only explanation at hand of this relative superiority of brain weight in old women is that with the close of the period of reproduction (the anabolic surplus being no longer consumed in the processes associated with reproduction) the constructive tendency still asserts itself, and a slight access of growth and vitality results to the organism.

It must be confessed that the testimony of anthropologists on the difference in variability of men and women is to be accepted with great caution. As a class they have gone on the assumption that woman is an inferior creation, and have almost totally neglected to distinguish between the congenital characters of woman and those acquired as the result of a totally different relation to society on the part of women and men. They have also failed to appreciate the fact that differences from man are not necessarily points of inferiority, but adaptations to different and specialized modes of functioning. But, whatever may be the final interpretation of details, I think the evidence is sufficient to establish the following main propositions: Man consumes energy more rapidly; woman is more conservative of it. The structural variability of man is mainly toward motion; woman's variational tendency is not toward motion, but toward reproduction. Man is fitted for feats of strength and bursts of energy; woman has more stability and endurance. While woman remains nearer to the infantile type, man approaches more to the senile. The extreme variational tendency of man expresses itself in a larger percentage of genius, insanity, and idiocy; woman remains more nearly normal.

The fact that society is composed of two sexes, numerically almost equal, but differing in organic and social habits, is too significant to remain without influence on the structural and occupational sides of human life, and in the following chapters we shall note some of the influences of sex, and of the differences in bodily habit of men and women, on social forms and activities.

SEX AND PRIMITIVE SOCIAL CONTROL

The greater strength and restlessness of man and the more stationary condition of woman have a striking social expression in the fact that the earliest groupings of population were about the females rather than the males.

While at a disadvantage in point of force when compared with the male, the female has enjoyed a negative superiority in the fact that her sexual appetite was not so sharp as that of the male. Primitive man, when he desired a mate, sought her. The female was more passive and stationary. She exercised the right of choice, and had the power to transfer her choice more arbitrarily than has usually been recognized; but the need of protection and assistance in providing for offspring inclined her to a permanent union, and doubtless natural selection favored the groups in which parents co-operated in caring for the offspring. But assuming a relation permanent enough to be called marriage, the man was still, as compared with the woman, unsettled and unsocial. He secured food by violence or cunning, and hunting and fighting were fit expressions of his somatic habit.

The woman was the social nucleus, the point to which he returned from his wanderings. In this primitive stage of society, however, the bond between woman and child was altogether more immediate and constraining than the bond between woman and man. The maternal instinct is reinforced by necessary and constant association with the child. We can hardly find a parallel for the intimacy of association between mother and child during the period of lactation; and, in the absence of domesticated animals or suitable foods, and also, apparently, from simple neglect formally to wean the child, this connection is greatly prolonged. The child is frequently suckled from four to five years, and occasionally from ten to twelve.[95] In consequence we find society literally growing up about the woman. The mother and her children, and her children's children, and so on indefinitely in the female line, form a group. But the men were not so completely incorporated in this group as the women, not only because parentage was uncertain and naming of children consequently on the female side, but because the man was neither by necessity nor disposition so much a home-keeper as the women and their children.

The tangential disposition of the male is expressed in the system of exogamy so characteristic of tribal life. The movement toward exogamy doubtless originates in the restlessness of the male, the tendency to make new co-ordinations, the stimulus to seek more unfamiliar women, and the emotional interest in making unfamiliar sexual alliances. But, quite aside from its origin, exogamy is an energetic expression of the male nature. Natural selection favors the process by sparing the groups which by breeding out have heightened their physical vigor.[96] There results from this a social condition which, from the standpoint of modern ideas, is very curious. The man makes, and, by force of convention, finally must make, his matrimonial alliances only with women of other groups; but the woman still remains in her own group, and the children are members of her group, while the husband remains a member of his own clan, and is received, or may be received, as a guest in the clan of his wife. Upon his death his property is not shared by his children, nor by his wife, since these are not members of his clan; but it falls to the nearest of kin within his clan— usually to his sister's children.

The maternal system of descent is found in all parts of the world where social advance stands at a certain level, and the evidence warrants the assumption that every group which advances to a culture state passes through this stage. Morgan gives an account of this system among the Iroquois:

> Each household was made up on the principle of kin. The married women, usually sisters, own or collateral, were of the same gens or clan, the symbol or totem of which was often painted upon the house, while their husbands and the wives of their sons belonged to several other gentes. The children were of the gens of their mother. While husband and wife belonged to different gentes, the predominating number in each household would be of the same gens, namely, that of their mothers. As a rule the sons brought home their wives, and in some cases the husbands of the daughters were admitted to the maternal household. Thus each household was composed of a mixture

of persons of different gentes, but this would not prevent the numerical ascendency of the particular gens to whom the house belonged. In a village of one hundred and twenty houses, as the Seneca village of Tiotohatton described by Mr. Greenbalge in 1677, there would be several houses belonging to each gens. It presented a general picture of the Indian life in all parts of America at the epoch of European discovery.[97]

Morgan also quotes Rev. Ashur Wright, for many years a missionary among the Senecas and familiar with their language and customs:

As to their family system, when occupying the old log houses, it is probable that some one clan predominated, the women taking in husbands, however, from the other clans, and sometimes for novelty, some of their sons bringing in their young wives until they felt brave enough to leave their mothers. Usually the female portion ruled the house, and were doubtless clannish enough about it. The stores were in common, but woe to the luckless husband or lover who was too shiftless to do his share of the providing. No matter how many children or whatever goods he might have in the house, he might at any time be ordered to pick up his blanket and budge, and after such orders it would not be healthful for him to attempt to disobey; the house would become too hot for him, and, unless saved by the intercession of some aunt or grandmother, he must retreat to his own clan, or, as was often done, go and start a new matrimonial alliance in some other. The women were the great power among the clans as everywhere else. They did not hesitate, when occasion required, to "knock off the horns," so it was technically called, from the head of a chief and send him back to the ranks of the warriors. The original nomination of the chiefs, also, always rested with them.[98]

Traces of the maternal system are everywhere found on the American continent, and in some regions it is still in force. McGee says of the Seri stock of the southwest coast, now reduced to a single tribe, that the claims of a suitor are pressed by his female relatives, and, if the suit is favorably regarded by the mother and uncles of the girl, the suitor is provisionally installed in the house, without purchase price and presents. He is then expected to show his worthiness of a permanent relation by demonstrating his ability as a provider, and by showing himself an implacable foe to aliens. He must support all the female relatives of his bride's family by the products of his skill and industry in hunting and fishing for a year. He is the general protector of the girl's family, and especially of the girl, whose bower and pelican-skin couch he shares, "not as husband, but as continent companion," for a year. If all goes well, he is then permanently received as "consort-guest," and his children are added to the clan of his mother-in-law.[99] With few exceptions, descent was formerly reckoned in Australia in the female line, and the usage survives in some regions. Howitt, in a letter to Professor Tylor, reports of the tribes near Maryborough, Queensland:

> When a man marries a woman from a distant locality, he goes to her tribelet and identifies himself with her people. This is a rule with very few exceptions. Of course, I speak of them as they were in their wild state. He becomes a part of, and one of, the family. In the event of a war expedition, the daughter's husband acts as a blood-relation, and will fight and kill his own blood-relations, if blows are struck by his wife's relations. I have seen a father and son fighting under these circumstances, and the son would most certainly have killed the father, if others had not interfered.[100]

In Australia there is also a very sharp social expression of the fact of sex in the division of the group into male and female classes in addition to the division into clans.[101] In the Malay Archipelago the same system is found.

> Among the Padang Malays the child always belongs to its mother's *suku*, and all blood-relationship is reckoned through the wife as the real transmitter of the family, the husband being only a stranger. For this reason his heirs are not his own children, but the children of his sister, his brothers, and other uterine relations; children are the natural heirs of their mother only…. We may assume that, wherever exogamy is now found coexisting with inheritance through the father (as among Rejangs and Bataks, the people of Nias and Timor, or the Alfurs of Ceram and Buru), this was formerly through the mother; and that the other system has grown up out of dislike to the inconveniences arising

from the insecure and dependent condition of the husband in the wife's family.[102]

In Africa descent through females is the rule, with exceptions. The practice of the Wamoima, where the son of the sister is preferred in legacies, because "a man's own son is only the son of his wife," is typical.[103] Battel reported that the state of Loango was ruled by four princes, the sons of the former king's sister, since the own sons of the king never succeeded.[104]

Traces of this system are found in China and Japan, and it is still in full force in parts of India. Among the Kasias of northeast India the husband resides in the house of his wife, or visits her occasionally.

> Laws of rank and property follow the strictest maternal type; when a couple separate, the children remain with the mother; the son does not succeed his father, but the raja's neglected offspring may become a common peasant or laborer; the sister's son succeeds to rank, and is heir to the property.[105]

Male kinship prevails among the Arabs, but Professor Robertson Smith has discovered abundant evidence that the contrary practice prevailed in ancient Arabia.

> The women of the Jâhilîya, or some of them, had the right to dismiss their husbands, and the form of dismissal was this: If they lived in a tent, they turned it round, so that, if the door had faced east, it now faced west, and when the man saw this, he knew that he was dismissed, and did not enter.[106]

And after the establishment of the male system the women still held property—a survival from maternal times. A form of divorce pronounced by a husband was, "Begone! for I will no longer drive thy flocks to the pasture."[107]

> Our evidence seems to show that, when something like regular marriage began, and a free tribeswoman had one husband or one

definite group of husbands at a time, the husbands at first came to her and she did not go to them.[108]

Numerous survivals of the older system are also found among the Hebrews. The servant of Abraham anticipated that the bride whom he was sent to bring for Isaac might be unwilling to leave her home, and the presents which he carried went to Rebekah's mother and brother.[109] Laban says to Jacob, "These daughters are my daughters, and these children are my children;"[110] the obligation to blood-vengeance rests apparently on the maternal kindred;[111] Samson's Philistine wife remained among her people;[112] and the injunction in Gen. 2:24, "Therefore shall a man leave his father and his mother, and shall cleave unto his wife," refers to the primitive Hebraic form of marriage.[113] Where the matriarchate prevails we naturally find no prejudice against marriage with a half-sister on the father's side, while union with a uterine sister is incestuous. Sara was a half-sister of Abraham on the father's side, and Tamar could have married her half-brother Amnon,[114] though they were both children of David; and a similar condition prevailed in Athens under the laws of Solon.[115] Herodotus says of the Lycians:

> Ask a Lycian who he is, and he will answer by giving his own name, that of his mother, and so on in the female line. Moreover, if a free woman marry a man who is a slave, their children are free citizens; but if a free man marry a foreign woman, or cohabit with a concubine, even though he be the first person in the state, the children forfeit all rights of citizenship.[116]

Herodotus also relates that when Darius gave to the wife of Intaphernes permission to claim the life of a single man of her kindred, she chose her brother, saying that both husband and children could be replaced.[117] The declaration of Antigone in Sophocles,[118] that she would have performed for neither husband nor children the toil which she undertook for Polynices, against the will of the citizens, indicates that the tie of a common womb was stronger than the social tie of marriage. The extraordinary honor, privilege, and proprietary rights enjoyed by ancient Egyptian and Babylonian wives[119] are traceable to an earlier maternal organization.

All ethnologists admit that descent through females has been very widespread, but some deny that this system has been universally prevalent at any stage of culture. Those who have diminished its importance, however, have done so chiefly in reinforcement of their denials of the theory of promiscuity. It has been very generally assumed that maternal descent is due solely to uncertainty of paternity, and that an admission that the maternal system has been universal is practically an admission of promiscuity. Opponents of this theory have consequently felt called upon to minimize the importance of maternal descent.[120] But descent through females is not, in fact, fully explained by uncertainty of parentage on the male side. It is due to the larger social fact, including this biological one, that the bond between mother and child is the closest in nature, and that the group grew up about the more stationary female; and consequently the questions of maternal descent and promiscuity are by no means so inseparable as has commonly been assumed. We may accept Sir Henry Maine's terse remark that "paternity is a matter of inference, as opposed to maternity, which is a matter of observation,"[121] without concluding that society would have been first of all patriarchal in organization, even if paternity had been also a matter of observation. For the association of the woman with the child is immediate and perforce, but the immediate interest of the man is in the woman, through the power of her sexual attractiveness, and his interest in the child is secondary and mediated through her. This relation being a constant one, having its roots in the nature of sex rather than in the uncertainty of parentage, we may safely conclude that the so-called "mother-right" has everywhere preceded "father-right," and was the fund from which the latter was evolved.

But while it is natural that the children and the group should grow up about the mother, it is not conceivable that woman should definitely or long control the activities of society, especially on their motor side. In view of his superior power of making movements and applying force, the male must inevitably assume control of the life direction of the group, no matter what the genesis of the group. It is not a difficult conclusion that, if woman's leaping, lifting, running, climbing, and slugging capacity is inferior to man's, by however slight a margin, her fighting capacity is less in the same degree; for battle is only an application of force, and there has never been a moment in the history of society when the law of might, tempered by sexual affinity, did not prevail. We must then, in fact, recognize a sharp distinction between the law of descent and the fact of authority.

The male was everywhere present in primitive society, and everywhere made his force felt. We can see this illustrated most plainly in the animal group, where the male is the leader, by virtue of his strength. There is also a stage of human society which may be called the prematriarchal stage, from the fact that ideas of kinship are so feeble that no extensive social filiation is effected through this principle, in consequence of which the group has not reached the tribal stage of organization on the basis of kinship, but remains in the primitive biological relation of male, female, and offspring. The Botocudos, Fuegians, Eskimos, West Australians, Bushmen, and Veddahs represent this primitive stage more or less completely; they have apparently not reached the stage where the fact of kinship expresses itself in maternal organization. They live in scattered bands, held together loosely by convenience, safety, and inertia, and the male is the leader; but the leadership of the male in this case, as among animals, is very different from the organized and institutional expression of the male force in systems of political control growing out of achievement. This involves a social history through which these low tribes have not passed.

Organization cannot proceed very far in the absence of social mass, and the collection of social mass took place unconsciously about the female as a universal preliminary of the conscious synthetization of the mass through males. From the side of organization, the negative accretion of population about female centers and filiation through blood is very precious, since filiation based on relation to females prepares the way for organization based on motor activities.[122] But in the prematernal stage, in the maternal stage, and in the patriarchal stage the male force was present and was the carrier of the social will. In the fully maternal system, indeed, the male authority is only thinly veiled, or not at all. Filiation through female descent precedes filiation through achievement, because it is a function of somatic conditions, in the main, while filiation through achievement is a function of historical conditions. This advantage of maternal organization in point of time embarrasses and obscures the individual and collective expression of the male force, but under the veil of female nomenclature and in the midst of the female organization we can always detect the presence of the male authority. Bachofen's conception of the maternal system as a political system was erroneous, as Dargun and others have pointed out,[123] though woman has been reinforced by the fact of descent, and has so figured somewhat in political systems.

A most instructive example of the parallel existence of descent through females and of male authority is found in the Wyandot tribe of Indians, in which also the participation of woman in the regulative activities of society is, perhaps, more systematically developed than in any other single case among maternal peoples. Major Powell gives the following outline of the civil and military government of this tribe:

> The civil government inheres in a system of councils and chiefs. In each gens there is a council, composed of four women, called *Yu-waí-yu-wá-na*. These four women councilors select a chief of the gens from its male members—that is, from their brothers and sons. This gentile chief is the head of the gentile council. The council of the tribe is composed of the aggregated gentile councils. The tribal council, therefore, is composed one-fifth of men and four-fifths of women. The sachem of the tribe, or tribal chief, is chosen by the chiefs of the gentes. There is sometimes a grand council of the gens, composed of the councilors of the gens proper and all the heads of households (women) and leading men—brothers and sons. There is also a grand council of the tribe, composed of the council of the tribe proper and the heads of households of the tribe, and all the leading men of the tribe....

> The four women councilors of the gens are chosen by the heads of households, themselves being women. There is no formal election, but frequent discussion is had over the matter from time to time, in which a sentiment grows up within the gens and throughout the tribe that, in the event of the death of any councilor, a certain person will take her place. In this manner there are usually one, two, or more potential councilors in each gens, who are expected to attend all the meetings of the council, though they take no part in the deliberations and have no vote. When a woman is installed as a councilor, a feast is prepared by the gens to which she belongs, and to this feast all the members of the

tribe are invited. The woman is painted and dressed in her best attire, and the sachem of the tribe places upon her head the gentile chaplet of feathers, and announces in a formal manner to the assembled guests that the woman has been chosen a councilor.... The gentile chief is chosen by the council women after consultation with the other women and men of the gens. Often the gentile chief is a potential chief through a period of probation. During this time he attends the meetings of the council, but takes no part in the deliberations and has no vote. At his installation, the council women invest him with an elaborately ornamented tunic, place upon his head a chaplet of feathers, and paint the gentile totem upon his face.... The sachem of the tribe is selected by the men belonging to the council of the tribe.

The management of military affairs inheres in the military council and chief. The military council is composed of all the able-bodied men of the tribe; the military chief is chosen by the council from the Porcupine gens. Each gentile chief is responsible for the military training of the youth under his authority. There are usually one or more potential military chiefs, who are the close companions and assistants of the chief in time of war and, in case of the death of the chief, take his place in the order of seniority.[124]

In this tribe the numerical recognition of women is striking, and indicates that they are the original core of society. They are still responsible for society, in a way, but all the offices involving motor activity are deputed to men. Thus women, as heads of households, choose four women councilors of the clan (gens), and these choose the fifth member, who is a man and the head of the council and chief of the clan. The tribal chief is, however, chosen by males, and in the military organization, which represents the group capacity for violence, the women have not even a nominal recognition. The real authority rests with those who are most fit to exercise it. Female influence persists as a matter of habit, until, under the pressure of social, particularly of military, activities, the breaking-up of the habit and a new accommodation follows the accumulation of a larger fund of social energy.

The men of any group are at any time in possession of the force to change the habits of the group and push aside any existing system. But the savage is not revolutionary; his life and his social sanctions are habitual. He is averse to change as such, and retains form and rite after their meaning is lost. We consequently find an expression of social respect for woman under the maternal system suggestive of chivalry, and even a formal elevation of women to authority in groups where the actual control is in the hands of men.

In the Mariana Islands the position of woman was distinctly superior; even when the man had contributed an equal share of property on marriage, the wife dictated everything and the man could undertake nothing without her approval; but, if the woman committed an offense, the man was held responsible and suffered the punishment. The women could speak in the assembly, they held property, and if a woman asked anything of a man, he gave it up without a murmur. If a wife was unfaithful, the husband could send her home, keep her property, and kill the adulterer; but if the man was guilty, or even suspected of the same offense, the women of the neighborhood destroyed his house and all his visible property, and the owner was fortunate if he escaped with a whole skin; and if a wife was not pleased with her husband, she withdrew, and a similar attack followed. On this account many men were not married, preferring to live with paid women. Likewise, in the Gilbert Islands a man shows the same respect to a woman as to a chief, by stepping aside when he meets her. If a man strikes a woman, the other women drive him from the tribe. On Lukunor the men used, in conversation with women, not the usual, but a deferential form of language.[125]

The discoverers of the Friendly Islands found there a king in authority over the people, and his wife in control of the king, receiving homage from him, but not ruling.[126] In these and similar cases woman's early relation to the household is formally retained in the larger group and in the presence of an obviously masculine form of organization.

But, in contrast with the survival in political systems of the primitive respect shown mothers, we find the assertion of individual male force within the very bosom of the maternal organization, in the person of the husband, brother, or uncle of the woman. Among the Caribs "the father or head of the household exerts unlimited authority over his wives and children, but this authority is not founded on legal rights, but upon his physical superiority."[127] In spite of the maternal system in North America, the women were often roughly handled by their husbands. Schoolcraft says of the Kenistenos: "When a young man marries, he immediately goes to live with the father and mother of his wife, who treat him, nevertheless, as an entire stranger till after the birth of his first child." But

> it appears that chastity is considered by them as a virtue ... and it sometimes happens that the infidelity of a wife is punished by the husband with the loss of her hair, nose, or perhaps life. Such severity proceeds, perhaps, less from rigidity of virtue than from its having been practiced without his permission; for a temporary interchange of wives is not uncommon, and the offer of their persons is considered as a necessary part of the hospitality due to strangers.[128]

Schoolcraft also says of the women of the Chippeways, among whom the maternal system had given way:

> They are very submissive to their husbands, who have however, their fits of jealousy; and for very trifling causes treat them with such cruelty as sometimes to occasion their death. They are frequently objects of traffic, and the father possesses the right of disposing of his daughter.[129]

Indian fathers also frequently sold their children, without any show of right. "Kane mentions that the Shastas ... frequently sell their children as slaves to the Chinooks."[130] Bancroft says of the Columbians: "Affection for children is by no means rare, but in few tribes can they resist the temptation to sell or gamble them away."[131] Descent through mothers is in force among the negroes of equatorial Africa, the man's property passing to his sister's children; but the father is an unlimited despot, and no one dares to oppose him. So long as his relation with his wives continues, he is master of them and of their children. He can even sell the latter into slavery.[132] In New Britain maternal descent prevails, but wives are obtained by purchase or capture, and are practically slaves; they are cruelly treated, carry on agriculture, and bear burdens which make them prematurely stooped, and are likely, if their husbands are offended, to be killed and eaten.[133]

In many regions of Australia women are treated with extreme brutality, when their work is not satisfactory, or the husband has any other cause for offense. In Victoria the men often break their staves over the heads of the women, and skulls of women have been found in which knitted fractures indicated former ill-treatment. In Cape York the women are beaten, and in the interior an angry native burned his wife alive. In the Adelaide dialect the phrase "owner of a woman" means husband. When a man dies, his uterine brother inherits his wife and children.[134]

Where under an exogamous system of marriage a man is forced to go outside his group to obtain a wife, he may do this either by going over to her group, by taking possession of her violently, or by offering her and the members of her group sufficient inducements to relinquish her; and the contrasted male and female disposition is expressed in all the forms of marriage incident to the exogamous system. Every exogamous group is naturally reluctant to relinquish its women, both because it has in them laborers and potential mothers whose children will be added to the group, and because, in the event of their remaining in the group after marriage, their husbands become additional defenders and providers within the group. Where the husband is to settle in the family of the wife, a test is consequently often made of his ability as a provider. Among the Zuni Indians there is no purchase price, no general exchange of gifts; but as soon as the agreement is reached, the young man must undertake certain duties:

He must work in the field of his prospective mother-in-law, that his strength and industry may be tested; he must collect fuel and deposit it near the maternal domicile, that his disposition as a provider may be made known; he must chase and slay the deer, and make from an entire buckskin a pair of moccasins for the bride, and from other skins and textiles a complete feminine suit, to the end that his skill in hunting, skin-dressing, and weaving may be displayed; and, finally, he must fabricate or obtain for the maiden's use a necklace of seashell or of silver, in order that his capacity for long journeys or successful barter may be established; but if circumstances prevent him from performing these duties actually, he may perform them symbolically, and such performance is usually acceptable to the elder people. After these preliminaries are completed, he is formally adopted by his wife's parents, yet remains merely a perpetual guest, subject to dislodgment at his wife's behest, though he cannot legally withdraw from the covenant; if dissatisfied, he can only so ill-treat his wife or children as to compel his expulsion.[135]

This practice is seen in a symbolical form where presents are required of the suitor before marriage and their equivalent returned later. By depositing goods accumulated through his activities he demonstrates his ability as a provider, without undergoing a formal test. This practice is reported of the Indians of Oregon:

The suitor never, in person, asks the parents for their daughter; but he sends one or more friends, whom he pays for their services. The latter sometimes effect their purposes by feasts. The offer generally includes a statement of the property which will be given for the wife to the parents, consisting of horses, blankets, or buffalo robes. The wife's relations always raise as many horses (or other property) for her dower as the bridegroom has sent the parents, but scrupulously take care not to turn over the same horses or the same articles.... This is the custom alike of the Walla-Wallas, Nez-Percés, Cayuse, Waskows, Flatheads, and Spokanes.[136]

In Patagonia the usual custom is for the bridegroom, after he has secured the consent of his damsel, to send either a brother or some intimate friend to the parents, offering so many mares, horses, or silver ornaments for the bride. If the parents consider the match desirable, as soon after as circumstances will permit, the bridegroom, dressed in his best, and mounted on his best horse, proceeds to the toldo of his intended, and hands over the gifts; the parents then return gifts of equivalent value, which, however, in the event of a separation are the property of the bride.[137]

Marriage by capture is an immediate expression of male force. Like marriage by settlement in the house of the wife, it is an expedient for obtaining a wife outside the group where marriage by purchase is not developed, or where the suitor cannot offer property for the bride. It is an unsocial procedure and does not persist in a growing society, for it involves retaliation and blood-feud. But it is a desperate means of avoiding the constraint and embarrassment of a residence in the family and among the relatives of the wife, where the power of the husband is hindered, and the male disposition is not satisfied in this matter short of personal ownership.

The man also sometimes lives under the maternal system in regular marriage, but escapes its disadvantages by stealing a supplementary wife or purchasing a slave woman, over whom and whose children he has full authority. In the Babar Archipelago, where the maternal system persists, even in the presence of marriage by purchase (the man living in the house of the woman, and the children reckoned with the mother), it is considered highly honorable to steal an additional wife from another group, and in this case the children belong to the father.[138] Among the Kinbundas of Africa children belong to the maternal uncle, who has the right to sell them, while the father regards as his children in fact the offspring of a slave woman, and these he treats as his personal property. To the same effect, among the Wanyamwesi, south of the Victoria Nyanza, the children of a slave wife inherit, to the exclusion of children born of a legal wife. And husbands among the Fellatahs are in the habit of adopting children, though they may have sons or daughters of their own, and the adopted children inherit the property.[139] In Indonesia a man sometimes marries a woman and settles in her family, and the children belong to her. But he may later carry her forcibly to his own group, and the children then belong to him.[140]

Bosman relates that in Guinea religious symbolism was also introduced by the husband to reinforce and lend dignity to this action. The maternal system held with respect to the chief wife:

> It was customary, however, for a man to buy and take to wife a slave, a friendless person with whom he could deal at pleasure, who had no kindred that could interfere for her, and to consecrate her to his Bossum or god. The Bossum wife, slave as she had been, ranked next to the chief wife, and was like her exceptionally treated. She alone was very jealously guarded, she alone was sacrificed at her husband's

death. She was, in fact, wife in a peculiar sense. And having, by consecration, been made of the kindred and worship of her husband, her children would be born of his kindred and worship.[141]

Altogether the most satisfactory means of removing a girl from her group is to purchase her. The use of property in the acquisition of women is not a particular expression of the male nature, since property is accumulated by females as well; but where this form of marriage exists it means practically that the male relatives of the girl are using her for profit, and that her suitor is seeking more complete control of her than he can gain in her group; and viewed in this light the purchase and sale of women is an expression of the dominant nature of the male. In consequence of purchase, woman became in barbarous society a chattel, and her socially constrained position in history and the present hindrances to the outflow of her activities are to be traced largely to the system of purchasing wives.

The simplest form of purchase is to give a woman in exchange. "The Australian male almost invariably obtains his wife or wives either as the survivor of a married elder brother or in exchange for his sisters, or, later in life, for his daughters."[142] A wife is also often sold on credit, but kept at home until the price is paid. On the island of Serang a youth belongs to the family of the girl, living according to her customs and religion until the bride-price is paid. He then takes both wife and children to his tribe. But in case he is very poor, he never pays the price, and remains perpetually in the tribe of his wife.[143] Among the Kwakiutl Indians of British Columbia the maternal has only barely given way to the paternal system, and the form of marriage reflects both systems. The suitor sends a messenger with blankets, and the number sent is doubled within three months, making in all about one hundred and fifty. These are to be returned later. He is then allowed to live with the girl in her father's house. Three months later the husband gives perhaps a hundred blankets more for permission to take his wife home.[144] Among the Makassar and Beginese stems of Indionesia the purchase of a wife involves only a partial relinquishment of the claim of the maternal house on the girl; the purchase price is paid by instalments and all belongs to the mother's kindred in case full payment is not made. A compromise between the two systems is made on the Molucca Islands, where children born before the bride-price is paid belong to the mother's side, after that to the father's.[145]

So long as a wife remained in her group, she could rely upon her kindred for protection against ill-usage from her husband, but she forfeited this advantage when she passed to his group. An Arabian girl replies to her father, when a chief seeks her in marriage: "No! I am not fair of face, and I have infirmities of temper, and I am not his *bint'amm* (tribeswoman), so that he should respect my consanguinity with him, nor does he dwell in thy country, so that he should have regard for thee; I fear then that he may not care for me and may divorce me, and so I shall be in an evil case."[146] The Hassanyeh Arabs of the White Nile region in Egypt afford a curious example of the conflict of male and female interests in connection with marriage, in which the female passes by contract for only a portion of her time under the authority of the male:

> When the parents of the man and woman meet to settle the price of the woman, the price depends on how many days in the week the marriage tie is to be strictly observed. The woman's mother first of all proposes that, taking everything into consideration, with a due regard for the feelings of the family, she could not think of binding her daughter to a due observance of that chastity which matrimony is expected to command for more than two days in the week. After a great deal of apparently angry discussion, and the promise on the part of the relatives of the man to pay more, it is arranged that the marriage shall hold good, as is customary among the first families of the tribe, for four days in the week, viz.: Monday, Tuesday, Wednesday, and Thursday; and, in compliance with old-established custom, the marriage rites during the three remaining days shall not be insisted on, during which days the bride shall be perfectly free to act as she may think proper, either by adhering to her husband and home, or by enjoying her freedom and independence from all observation of matrimonial obligations.[147]

We may understand also that the tolerance of loose conduct in girls before marriage—a tolerance which amounts in many tribes to approval—is due to the tribal recognition of the value of children, and children born out of marriage are added to the family of the mother. When, on the other hand, the conduct of the girl is strictly watched, this is from a consideration that virgins command a higher bride-price. Child-marriages and long betrothals are means of guaranteeing the proper conduct of a girl to her husband, as they constitute a personal claim and afford him an opportunity to throw more restrictions about her. So that, in any case, the conduct of the girl is viewed with reference to her value to the tribe.

A social grouping which is not the product of forces more active in their nature than the reproductive force may be expected to yield before male motor activities, when these are for any reason sufficiently formulated. The primitive warrior and hunter comes into honor and property through a series of movements involving judgments of time and space, and the successful direction of force, aided by mechanical appliances and mediated through the hand and the eye. Whether directed against the human or the animal world, the principle is the same; success and honor and influence in tribal life depend on the application of violence at the proper time, in the right direction, and in sufficient measure; and this is pre-eminently the business of the male. The advantage of acting in concert in war and hunting, and under the leadership of those who have shown evidence of the best judgment in these matters, is felt in any body of men who are held together by any tie; and the first tie is the tie of blood, by which we should understand, not that primitive man has any sentimental feeling about kinship, but that he is psychologically inseparable from those among whom he was born and with whom he has to do. Though the father's sense of kinship and interest in his children is originally feeble, it increases with the growth of consciousness in connection with various activities, and, at the point in race development when chieftainship is hereditary in the clan and personal property is recognized, the father realizes the awkwardness of a social system which reckons his children as members of another clan and forces him to bequeath his rank and possessions to his sister's children, or other members of his own group, rather than to his children. The Navajoes[148] and Nairs,[149] and ancient Egyptians[150] avoided this unpleasant condition by giving their property to their children during their own lifetime; and the Shawnees, Miamis, Sauks, and Foxes avoided it by naming the children into the clan of the father, giving a child a tribal name being equivalent to adoption.[151] The cleverest bit of primitive politics of which we have record is the device employed in ancient Peru, and surviving in historical times in Egypt and elsewhere in the East, by which the ruler married his own sister, contrary to the exogamous practice of the common folk. The children might then be regularly reckoned as of the kin of the mother, indeed, but they were at the same time of and in the group of the father, and the king secured the succession of his own son by marrying the woman whose son would traditionally succeed.

As we should expect, the desirability of modifying the system of descent and inheritance through females is felt first in connection with situations of honor and profit. At the time of the discovery of the Hawaiian Islands the government was a brutal despotism, presenting many of the features of feudalism; the people prostrated themselves before the king and before objects which he had touched, and a man suffered death whose shadow fell upon the king, or who went uncovered within the shadow of the king's house, or even looked upon the king by day.[152] But descent was in the female line, with a tendency to transfer to the male line in case of the king, and among chiefs, priests, and nobility.[153] This assertion of the male authority was sometimes resented, however, and was a source of frequent trouble. Wilkes states that there was formerly no regularly established order of succession to the throne; the children of the chief wife had the best claim, but the king often named his own successor, and this gave rise to violent conflicts.[154]

Blood-brotherhood, blood-vengeance, secret societies, tribal marks (totemism, circumcision, tattooing, scarification), and religious dedication are devices by which, consciously or unconsciously, the men escape from the tyranny of the maternal system. We cannot assume that these practices originate solely or largely in dissatisfaction, for the men would feel the advantage of a combination of interests whenever brought into association with one another; but these artificial bonds and their display to the eye are among the first attempts to synthetize the male forces of the group, and it is quite apparent that such unions are unfavorable to the continuance of the influence of women and of the system which they represent. In West Africa and among some of the negro tribes the initiatory ceremony is apparently deliberately hostile to the maternal organization. The youth is taken from the family of his mother, symbolically killed and buried, resurrected by the priests into a male organization, and dedicated to his father's god.[155]

Spatial conditions have played an important rôle also in the development of societies. Through movements the individual or the group is able to pick and choose advantageous relations, and by changing its location adjust itself to changes in the food conditions. That the success of the group is definitely related to its motor capacity is revealed by the following law of population, worked out by statisticians for the three predominant races of modern Europe: In countries inhabited jointly by these three races, the race possessing the smallest portion of wealth and the smallest representation among the more influential and educated classes constitutes also the least migratory element of the population, and tends in the least degree to concentrate in the cities and the more fertile regions of the country; and in countries inhabited jointly by the three races, the race possessing the largest portion of wealth and the largest representation among the more influential and educated classes is also the most migratory element of the population, and tends in the greatest degree to concentrate in the cities and the more fertile portions of the country.[156] The primitive movements of population necessitated by climatic change, geological disturbances, the failure of water or exhaustion of the sources of food, were occasions for the expression of the superior motor disposition of the male and for the dislodgment of the female from her position of advantage.

We know that the migrations of the natural races are necessary and frequent, and the movements of the culture races have been even more complex. The leadership of these mass-movements and spatial reaccommodations necessarily rests with the men, who, in their wanderings, have become acquainted with larger stretches of space; and whose specialty is motor co-ordination. The progressive races have managed the space problem best. At every favorable point they have pushed out their territorial boundaries or transferred their social activities to a region more favorable to their expansion. Under male leadership, in consequence, territory has always become the prize in every conflict of races; the modern state is based not on blood but on territory, and territory is at present the reigning political ideal.

In the process of coming into control of a larger environment through the motor activities of the male, the group comes into collision with other groups within which the same movement is going on, and it then becomes a question which group can apply force more destructively and remove or bring under control this human portion of its environment. Military organization and battle afford the grand opportunity for the individual and mass expression of the superior force-capacity of the male. They also determine experimentally which groups and which individuals are superior in this respect, and despotism, caste, slavery, and the subjection of women are concrete expressions of the trial.

The nominal headship of woman within the maternal group existed only in default of forms of activity fit to formulate headship among the men, and when chronic militancy developed an organization among the males, the political influence of the female was completely shattered. At a certain point in history women became an unfree class, precisely as slaves became an unfree class—because neither class showed a superior fitness on the motor side; and each class is regaining its freedom because the race is substituting other forms of decision for violence.

SEX AND SOCIAL FEELING

An examination of the early habits of man and an analysis of the instincts which persist in him show that he has been essentially a predaceous animal, fighting his way up at every step of the struggle for existence. It therefore becomes a point of considerable interest to determine what influences have contributed to soften his behavior and make it possible for him to dwell in harmony and co-operation with large groups of his fellows.

We, the lineal representatives of the successful enactors of one scene of slaughter after another, must, whatever more pacific virtues we may also possess, still carry about with us, ready to burst at any moment into flame, the smouldering and sinister traits of character by means of which they lived through so many massacres, harming others, but themselves unharmed.... If evolution and the survival of the fittest be true at all, the destruction of prey and of human rivals must have been among the most important of man's primitive functions, the fighting and the chasing instincts *must* have become ingrained. Certain perceptions *must* immediately, and without the intervention of inferences and ideas, have prompted emotions and motor discharges; and both the latter must, from the nature of the case, have been very violent, and therefore when unchecked of an intensely pleasurable

kind. It is just because bloodthirstiness is such a primitive part of us that it is so hard to eradicate, especially where a fight or a hunt is promised as a part of the fun.... No! those who try to account for this from above downwards, as if it resulted from the consequences of the victory being rapidly inferred, and from the agreeable sensations associated with them in the imagination, have missed the root of the matter. Our ferocity is blind and can only be explained from *below*. Could we trace it back through our lines of descent, we should see it taking more and more the form of a fatal reflex response, and at the same time becoming more and more the pure and direct emotion that it is.[157]

If we examine, in fact, our pleasures and pains, our moments of elation and depression, we find that they go back for the most part to instincts developed in the struggle for food and rivalry for mates. We can perhaps best get at the meaning of the conflict interest to the organism in terms of the significance to itself or the organism's own movements. Locomotion, of whatever type, is primarily to enable the animal to reach and grasp food, and also to escape other animals bent on finding food. The structure of the organism has been built up gradually through the survival of the most efficient structures. Corresponding with a structure mechanically adapted to successful movements, there is developed on the psychic side an interest in the conflict situation as complete and perfect as is the structure itself. The emotional states are, indeed, organic preparations for action, corresponding broadly with a tendency to advance or retreat, and a connection has even been made out between pleasurable states and the extensor muscles, and painful states and the flexor muscles. We can have no adequate idea of the time consumed and the experiments made in nature before the development of these types of structure and interest of the conflict pattern, but we know from the geological records that the time and experiments were long and many, and the competition so sharp, that finally, not in man alone, but in all the higher classes of animals, body and mind, structure and interest, were working perfectly in motor actions of the violent type involved in a life of conflict, competition, and rivalry. There could not have been developed an organism depending on offensive and defensive movements for food and life without an interest in what we call a dangerous or precarious situation. A type without this interest would have been defective, and would have dropped out in the course of development.

There has been comparatively little change in human structure or human interest in historical times. It is a popular view that moral and cultural views and interests have superseded our animal instincts; but the cultural period is only a span in comparison with prehistoric times and the prehuman period of life, and it seems probable that types of psychic reaction were once for all developed and fixed; and while objects of attention and interest in different historical periods are different, we shall never get far away from the original types of stimulus and reaction. It is, indeed, a condition of normal life that we should not get too far away from them.

The fact that our interests and enthusiasms are called out in situations of the conflict type is shown by a glance at the situations which arouse them most readily. War is simply an organized form of fight, and as such is most attractive, or, to say the least, arouses the interests powerfully. With the accumulation of property, and the growth of sensibility and intelligence, it becomes apparent that war is a wasteful and unsafe process, and public and personal interests lead us to avoid it as much as possible. But, however genuinely war may be deprecated, it is certainly an exciting game. The Rough Riders in this country recently, and more recently the young men of the aristocracy of England, went to war from motives of patriotism, no doubt; but there are unmistakable evidences that they also regarded it as the greatest sport they were likely to have a chance at in a lifetime. And there is evidence in plenty that the emotional attitude of women toward war is no less intense. Grey[158] relates that half a dozen old women among the Australians will drive the men to war with a neighboring tribe over a fancied injury. The Jewish maidens went out with music and dancing, and sang that Saul had slain his thousands, but David his ten thousands. Two American women who passed through the horrors of the siege of Pekin were, on their return, given a reception by their friends, and the daily press reported that they exhibited among other trophies "a Boxer's sword with the blood still on the blade, which was taken from the body of a Boxer killed by the legation guards; and a Boxer spear with which a native Christian girl was struck down in Legation Street." It is not necessary to regard as morbid or vulgar the action of these ladies in bringing home reminders of their peril. On the contrary, it is a sign of continued animal health and instinct in the race to feel deep interest in perilous situations and pleasure in their revival in consciousness.

"Unaccommodated man" was, to begin with, in relations more hostile than friendly. The struggle for food was so serious a fact, and predaceousness to such a degree the habit of life, that a suspicious, hostile, and hateful state of mind was the rule, with exceptions only in the cases where truce, association, and alliance had come about in the course of experience. This was still the state of affairs in so advanced a stage of development as the Indian society of North America, where a tribe was in a state of war with every tribe with which it had not made a treaty of peace; and it is perhaps true, generally speaking, of men today, that they regard others with a degree of distrust and aversion until they have proved themselves good fellows. What, indeed, would be the fate of a man on the streets of a city if he did otherwise? There has, nevertheless, grown up an intimate relation between man and certain portions of his environment; and this includes, not only his wife and children, his dog and his blood-brother, but, with lessening intensity, the members of his clan, tribe, and nation. These become, psychologically speaking, a portion of himself, and stand with him against the world at large. From the standpoint here outlined, prejudice or its analogue is the starting-point, and our question becomes one of the determination of the steps of the process by which man mentally allied with himself certain portions of his environment to the exclusion of others.

If we look for an explanation of the hostility which a group feels for another group, and of the sympathy which its members feel for one another, we may first of all inquire whether there are any conditions arising in the course of the biological development of a species which, aside from social activities, lead to a predilection for those of one's own kind and a prejudice against different groups. And we do, in fact, find such conditions. The earliest movements of animal life involve, in the rejection of stimulations vitally bad, an attitude which is the analogue of prejudice. On the principle of chemiotaxis, the micro-organism will approach a particle of food placed in the water and shun a particle of poison; and its movements are similarly controlled by heat, light, electricity, and other tropic forces.[159] The development of animal life from this point upward consists in the growth of structure and organs of sense adapted to discriminate between different stimulations, to choose between the beneficial and prejudicial, and to obtain in this way a more complete control of the environment. Passing over the lower forms of animal life, we find in the human type the power of attention, memory, and comparison highly developed, so that an estimate is put on stimulations and situations correspondent with the bearing of stimulations or situations of this type on welfare in the past. The choice and rejection involved in this process are accompanied by organic changes (felt as emotions) designed to assist in the action which follows a decision.[160] Both the judgment and the emotions are thus involved in the presentation to the senses of a situation or object involving possible advantage or hurt, pleasure or pain. It consequently transpires that the feelings called out on the presentation of disagreeable objects and their contrary are very different, and there arise in this connection fixed mental attitudes corresponding with fixed or habitually recurrent external situations—hate and love, prejudice and predilection—answering to situations which revive feelings of pain on the one hand, and feelings of pleasure on the other. And such is the working of suggestion that, not alone an object or situation may produce a given state of feeling, but a voice, an odor, a color, or any characteristic sign of an object may produce the same effect as the object itself. The sight or smell of blood is an excitant to a bull, because it revives a conflict state of feeling, and even the color of a red rag produces a similar effect.

When we come to examine in detail the process by which an associational and sympathetic relation is set up between the individual and certain parts of the outside world to the exclusion of others, we find this at first, on a purely instinctive and reflex basis, originating in connection with food-getting and reproduction, and growing more conscious in the higher forms of life. One of the most important origins of association and prepossession is seen in the relation of parents, particularly of mothers, to children. This begins, of course, among the lower animals. The mammalian class, in particular, is distinguished by the strength and persistence of the devotion of parents to offspring. The advantage secured by the form of reproduction characteristic of man and the other mammals is that a closer connection is secured between the child and the mother. By the intra-uterine form of reproduction the association of mother and offspring is set up in an organic way before the birth of the latter, and is continued and put on a social basis during the period of lactation and the early helpless years of the child. By continuing the helpless period of the young for a period of years, nature has made provision on the time side for a complex physical and mental type, impossible in types thrown at birth on their own resources. Along with the structural modification of the female on account of the intra-uterine form of reproduction and the effort of nature to secure a more complex type and a better chance of survival, there is a corresponding development of the sentiments, and maternal feeling, in particular, is developed as the subjective condition necessary to carrying out the plan of giving the infant a prolonged period of helplessness and play through which its faculties are developed.[161] The scheme would not work if the mother were not more interested in the child than in anything else in the world. In the course of development every variational tendency in mothers to dote on their children was rewarded by the survival of these children, and the consequent survival of the stock, owing to better nutrition, protection, and training. Of course, this inherited interest in children is shared by the males of the group also, though not in the same degree, and there is reason to believe also that the interest of the male parent in children is acquired in a great degree indirectly and socially through his more potent desire to associate with the mother.

This interest and providence on the score of offspring has also a characteristic expression on the mental side. All sense-perceptions are colored and all judgments biased where the child is in question, and affection for it extends to the particular marks which distinguish it. Not only its physical features, but its dress and little shoes, its toys and everything it has touched take on a peculiar aspect.

On the organic side, therefore, there is developed a tendency, both in connection with reactions to stimulations in general and in connection with reproductive life in particular, to seize on particular aspects and to be obsessed by them to the exclusion or disparagement of other aspects. The feelings of love and hate, and the broader feelings of race-prejudice and patriotism are consequently based first of all in the instincts.

Perhaps the most particular and interesting expression of the general fact of susceptibility is seen in the sensitiveness of man to the opinion in which he is held by others. Social life in every stage of society is characterized by an eagerness to make a striking effect. A bare reference to the ethnological facts in this connection will suffice: The Kite Indians have a society of young men so brave and so ostentatious of their bravery that they will not fight from cover nor turn aside to avoid running into an ambuscade or a hole in the ice. The African has the privilege of cutting a gash six inches long in his thigh for every man he has killed. The Melanesian who is planning revenge sets up a stick or stone where it can be seen; he refuses to eat, and stays away from the dance; he sits silent in the council and answers questions by whistling and by other signs draws attention to himself and has it understood that he is a brave and dangerous man, and that he is biding his time.[162]

This bidding for the good opinion of others has plainly a connection with food-getting, and with the conflict side of life. High courage is praised and valued by society, and a man of courage is less imposed on by others, and comes in for substantial recognition and the favor of women. It is thus of advantage to act in such a way as to get public approval and some degree of appreciation; and a degree of sensibility on the score of the opinion of others, or at least a reckoning upon this, is involved in the process of personal adjustment.

But the problem of personal adjustment at this point would seem to call for more of intelligence than emotion; and we find, on the contrary, an excess of sensibility and a mania for being well thought of hardly to be explained as originating in the exigencies of tribal organization, nor yet on the score of its service to the individual in getting his food and living out his life. Why could not primitive man live in society, be of the war-parties, plan ambuscades, develop his fighting technique and gear, be a blood-brother to another man, show his trophies, set a high value on his personality, and insist on recognition and respect, without this almost pathological dependence on the praise and blame of others?

Or if we approach the question from another standpoint and inspect our states of consciousness, we find signs that we have a greater fund of sensibility than is justified in immediate activity. We have the same mania to be well thought of; we are unduly interested when we hear that others have been talking about us; we are annoyed, even furious, at a slight criticism, and are childishly delighted by a compliment (without regard to our deserts); and children and adults alike understand how to put themselves forward and get notice, and equally well how to get notice by withdrawing themselves and staying away or out of a game. We have a tendency to show off which is not apparently genetically connected with exploit or organization, and we recognize that this form of vanity is not consistent with the ordinary run of our activities when we argue with ourselves that the opinion of this or that person is of no consequence and attempt to think ourselves into a state of indifference. Intellectually and deliberately our attitude toward criticism from others would often be, if we could choose, represented by Tweed's query: "What are you going to do about it?" But actually it puts us to bed.

All of this seems to indicate that there is an element in sensibility not accounted for on the exploit or food side, and this element is, I believe, genetically connected with sexual life. Unlike the struggle for existence in the ordinary sense of the phrase, the courtship of the sexes presents a situation in which an appeal is made for the favor of another personality, and the success of this appeal has a survival value—not for the individual, but for the species through the individual. We have, in fact, a situation in which the good opinion of another is vitally important. On this account the means of attracting and interesting others are definitely and bountifully developed among all the higher species of animals. Voice, plumage, color, odor, and movement are powerful excitants in wooing and aids both to the conquest of the female and the attraction of the male. In this connection we must also recognize the fact that reproductive life must be connected with violent stimulation, or it would be neglected and the species would become extinct; and, on the other hand, if the conquest of the female were too easy, sexual life would be in danger of becoming a play interest and a dissipation, destructive of energy and fatal to the species. Working, we may assume, by a process of selection and survival, nature has both secured and safeguarded reproduction. The female will not submit to seizure except in a high state of nervous excitation (as is seen especially well in the wooing of birds), while the male must conduct himself in such a way as to manipulate the female; and, as the more active agent, he develops a marvelous display of technique for this purpose. This is offset by the coyness and coquetry of the female, by which she equally attracts and fascinates the male and practices upon him to induce a corresponding state of nervous excitation.[163]

This is the only situation in the life of the lower animals, at any rate, where the choice of another is vitally important; and corresponding with the elaborate technique to secure this choice we have in wooing pleasure-pain reactions of a violent character. In a word, extreme sensitiveness to the judgment of another answers on the subjective side to technique for the conquest of a member of the opposite sex. It seems, therefore, that we are justified in concluding that our vanity and susceptibility have their origin largely in sexual life, and that, in particular, our susceptibility to the opinion of others and our dependence on their good will are genetically referable to sexual life.

This view would be completely substantiated if we could show that the qualities of vanity and susceptibility in question are present in any species where it is impossible to assume that they were developed in connection with the struggle for food and as the result of the survival of types showing a tendency to combine and co-operate in the effort to get food. And we do, in fact, have cases of this kind among some of the lower animals. It cannot be said that the dog, for instance, has survived in the struggle for existence because of his sensitiveness to public opinion in his species nor on account of an interest in being well thought of by the community of dogs at large which would lead him to behave in a public-spirited or moral manner. At the same time, the dog in his relation to man shows as keen a sensitiveness to man's opinion and treatment as does man himself. The attention which the master pays to one dog will almost break the heart of a dog not receiving it. A neglected dog plainly suffers as much in his way as the soldier who is sent to Coventry by his messmates; and if neglected and jealous dogs do not commit suicide, as they are reported to do, they are evidently in a state of mind to do so. This means that the dog has highly developed susceptibility to the appreciation of others, and that the species which he represents has had no history except a sexual history capable of developing this mental attitude. In connection with courtship he developed a fund of organic susceptibility, and this condition is involved in his more general relation to man; the machinery set up in sexual relations is played on by stimuli in general. A condition favorable to stimuli of a particular kind is favorable to stimuli in general; and it seems likely that this not very prominent fact of a state of excitation in a sexual connection is an important factor in the formation of the mind and of society.

There are also certain conditions in the development of the individual and of society where the sexual type of reaction is so near the surface that it shows through in connection with political, moral, and other essentially non-sexual activities. Passing over the fact that the period of adolescence is noticeably a period of "susceptibility" and personal vanity, we may take as an example of the intrusion or persistence of the sexual element in conditions of a non-sexual kind the frequent association of sexual with religious excitement.[164] The appeal made during a religious revival to an unconverted person has psychologically some resemblance to the attempt of the male to overcome the hesitancy of the female. In each case the will has to be set aside, and strong suggestive means are used; and in both cases the appeal is not of the conflict type, but of an intimate, sympathetic, and pleading kind. In the effort to make a moral adjustment, it consequently turns out that a technique is used which was derived originally from sexual life, and the use, so to speak, of the sexual machinery for a moral adjustment involves, in some cases, the carrying over into the general process of some sexual manifestations. The emotional forms used and the emotional states aroused are not entirely stripped of their sexual content.

On the race side, also, there is a stage in development where the sexual pattern is transferred almost unmodified to public affairs. The following extracts from a lengthy description given by Mr. Bowdich of his reception by the king of Ashanti, in the year 1817, will illustrate sufficiently the employment of the turkey-cock pattern of activity in political relations:

> The sun was reflected with a glare scarcely more supportable than the heat from massive gold ornaments which glistened in every direction. More than a hundred bands burst at once on our arrival, with the peculiar airs of their several chiefs; the horns flourished their defiances, with the beating of innumerable drums and metal instruments, and then yielded for a while to the soft breathings of their long flutes.... At least a hundred large umbrellas or canopies, which could shelter thirty persons, were sprung up and down by the bearers with brilliant effect, being made of scarlet, yellow, and the most showy cloths and silks, and crowned on the top with crescents, pelicans, elephants, barrels, and arms and swords of gold.... The caboceers, as did their superior captains, and attendants, wore Ashanti cloths of extravagant price, from the costly foreign silks which had been unravelled to weave them in all the varieties of color as well as pattern: they were of incredible size and weight, and thrown over the shoulder exactly like the Roman toga; a small silk fillet generally encircled their temples, and many gold necklaces, intricately wrought, suspended Moorish charms, dearly purchased, and enclosed in small square cases of gold, silver, and curious embroidery. Some wore necklaces reaching to the waist, entirely of aggry beads; a band of gold and beads encircled the knee, from which several strings of the same depended; small circlets of gold, like guineas, rings, and casts of animals were

strung round their ankles; their sandals were of green, red and delicate white leather; manillas, and rude lumps of rock gold hung from their left wrists, which were so heavily laden as to be supported on the head of one of their handsomest boys.... [The king] wore a fillet of aggry beads round his temples, a necklace of gold cockspur shells strung by their larger ends, and over his right shoulder a red silk cord, suspending three sapphires cased in gold; his bracelets were of the richest mixtures of beads and gold, and his fingers covered with rings; his cloth was of a dark green silk, a pointed diadem was elegantly painted in white on his forehead; also a pattern resembling an epaulette on each shoulder, and an ornament like a full blown rose, one leaf rising above another until it covered his whole breast.... The belts of the guards behind his chair were cased in gold, and covered with small jaw-bones of the same metal; the elephants' tails, waving like a small cloud before him, were spangled with gold, and large plumes of feathers were flourished among them. His eunuch presided over these attendants, wearing only one massive piece of gold about his neck; the royal stool, entirely cased in gold, was displayed under a splendid umbrella, with drums, sankos, horns, and various musical instruments, cased in gold, about the thickness of cartridge paper; large circles of gold hung by scarlet cloth from the swords of state;... hatchets of the same were intermixed with them; the breasts of the Ochras and various attendants were adorned with large stars, stools, crescents, and gossamer wings of solid gold.[165]

It is not surprising that the characteristically sexual method of display and emotional appeal should be associated with the earlier efforts at adjustment, both in the individual and in the state. This method is based on the instincts, and just as inhibition and brain legislation follow the instincts in point of development, a rational mode of control, individual and public, is developed later than the emotional form, or, at any rate, is not at first independent of it.

The origin of mental impressionability seems to lie then, not in one, but in the two general regions of activity—that connected with the struggle for food and that connected with reproduction. The strain on the attention in the food and conflict side of life involves the development of mental impressionability, particularly of an impressionability on the side of cognition. But in addition we have the impressionability growing out of sexual life which has been in question above, and which is more closely related to appreciation than to cognition. And of these two aspects of impressionability—the one growing out of conflict and the one growing out of reproduction—the latter has more social possibilities than the former, because it implies a sympathetic rather than an antagonistic organic attitude. It is certainly in virtue of susceptibility to the opinion of others that society works—through public opinion, fashion, tradition, reproof, encouragement, precept, and doctrine—to bring the individual under control and make him a member of society; and it is doubtful whether this could have been accomplished if a peculiar attitude of responsiveness to opinion had not arisen in sexual relations, reinforcing the more general and cognitive impressionability. Without this capacity to be influenced the individual would be in the condition of the hardened criminal, and society would be impossible.

This sex-susceptibility, which was originally developed as an accessory of reproduction and had no social meaning whatever, has thus, in the struggle of society to obtain a hold on the individual, become a social factor of great importance, and together with another product of sexual life—the love of offspring—it is, I suspect, the most immediate source of our sympathetic attitudes in general, and an important force in the development of the ideal, moral, and aesthetic sides of life.

Morality, sympathy, and altruism are of tribal origin, and have their roots in (1) the love of offspring, (2) the sensitivity connected with courtship, and (3) the comradeship which arises among men in prosecuting vital interests in common. The history of society on the moral and aesthetic sides is in great part the history of the attempt to make the sympathetic attitude prevail over the more antagonistic. But how far we are still short of this, and how far our sympathy and morality are still tribal and even familial, is indicated by the persistence of race-prejudice and of that

> lust in man no charm can tame
Of loudly publishing our neighbor's shame.

SEX AND PRIMITIVE INDUSTRY

Labor represents the expenditure of energy in securing food, and in making the food-process constant and sure; and we may well expect to find that the somatological differences shown to exist between man and woman will be found reflected in the labors of primitive society.

An examination of the ethnological facts shows that among the primitive races men are engaged in activities requiring strength, violence, speed, and the craft and foresight which follow from the contacts and strains of their more motor life; and the slow, unspasmodic, routine, stationary occupations are the part of woman. Animal life is itself motor, elusive, and violent, and both by disposition and of necessity man's attention and activities are devoted first of all to the animal process. It is the most stimulating and dangerous portion of his environment, and affords the most immediate and concrete reward.

Contrasted with this violent and intermittent activity of man, we find with equal uniformity that the attention of woman is directed principally to the vegetable environment. Man's attention to hunting and fighting, and woman's attention to agriculture and attendant stationary industries, is so generally a practice of primitive society that we may well infer the habit is based on a physiological difference. An explanation of exceptions to the rule, and the departure from it in the later life of the race, we shall have to seek in changes in the social habits of the race.

The old observation, that "woman was first a beast of burden, then a domestic animal, then a slave, then a servant, and last of all a minor," represents the usual view of the condition of woman taken by early missionaries and travelers. This view is, as we shall see, out of focus, but there is no doubt that the labors of early woman were exacting, incessant, varied, and hard, and that, if a catalogue of primitive forms of labor were made, woman would be found doing five things where man did one.

An Australian of the Kurnai tribe once said to Fison: "A man hunts, spears fish, fights, and sits about;"[166] and this is a very good general statement of the male activities of primitive society the world over, if we add one other activity—the manufacture of weapons. On the other hand, Bonwick's statement of the labors of Tasmanian women is a typical one:

> In addition to the necessary duty of looking after the children, they had to provide all the food for the household excepting that derived from the chase of the kangaroo. They climbed up hills for the opossum, delved in the ground with their sticks for yams, native bread, and nutritive roots, groped about the rocks for shellfish, dived beneath the sea for oysters, and fished for the finny tribe. In addition to this, they carried, on their frequent tramps, the household stuff in native baskets of their own manufacture. Their affectionate partners would even pile upon their burdens sundry spears and waddies not required for present service, and would command their help to rear the breakwind, and to raise the fire. They acted, moreover, as cooks to the establishment, and were occasionally regaled, at the termination of a feast, with the leavings of their gorged masters.[167]

Among the Andamanese, while the men go into the jungle to hunt pigs, the women fetch drinking water and firewood, catch shellfish, make fishing nets and baskets, spin thread, and cook the food ready for the return of the men.[168] In New Caledonia "girls work in the plantations, boys learn to fight."[169] In Africa the case is similar. Among the Bushmen (to take only one example from this continent) the woman "weaves the frail mats and rushes under which her family finds a little shelter from the wind and from the heat of the sun," constructs a fireplace of three round stones, fashions and bakes a few earthenware pots. When her household labors are done, she gathers roots, locusts, etc., from the fields. On the march she frequently carries a child, a mat, an earthen pot, some ostrich eggshells, and "a few ragged skins bundled on her head or shoulder," while the man carries only his spear, bow, and quiver.[170] The conditions among the American Indians were practically the same. Cotton Mather said of the Indians of Massachusetts: "The men are most abominably slothful, making their poor squaws or wives to plant, and dress, and barn, and beat their corn, and build their wigwams for them;"[171] and Jones, referring to the women of southern tribes, says:

> Doomed to perpetual drudgery and to that subordinate position to which woman is always consigned where civilization and religion are not, she was little less than a beast of burden, busy with cooking, the manufacture of pottery, mats, baskets, moccasins, etc., a tiller of the ground, a nurse for her own children, and at all times a servant to the commands and passions of the stronger sex.[172]

Primitive woman was therefore undoubtedly very busy, but I have seen no reason to believe that she considered her condition unfortunate. Our great-grandmothers were also very busy, but they were apparently not discontented. There was no reason why woman should not labor in primitive society. The forces which withdrew her from labor were expressions of later social conditions. Speaking largely, these considerations were the desire of men to preserve the beauty of women, and their desire to withdraw them from association with other men. It is the connection in thought and fact between idle and beautiful women and wealth, indeed, which has frequently led to the keeping of a superfluous number of such women as a sign of wealth.

The exemption of women from labor, in short, implied an economic surplus which early society did not possess. The lower classes of modern society do not possess it either, and there the women are still "drudges," if we want to use that word about a situation which is normal, in view of the economic condition of the men and women concerned. It was necessary that primitive society, in the absence of elaborate machinery for doing things, in unstable and precarious food conditions, and without resources accumulated from preceding generations, should utilize *all* its forces. The struggle for existence, in its harshest sense, was but little mitigated, and no group could have spared at all the industry of women. Even if primitive life had been as hard as Hobbes would have it, "solitary, poor, nasty, brutish, and short," mere negative, habitual hardness and miserableness of condition did not get the attention of primitive society particularly. Their life was hard, as we look at it, not as they looked at it. They could not compare themselves with the future, and comparisons with the past were doubtless in their favor. The best returns from activity will of course follow when each individual is doing something he is specially well fitted to do, and natural selection seems to have seen to it that primitive society should so divide the labor as best to utilize social energy by assigning to men the tasks requiring violent exertion, and to women those requiring constant attention.

But was not primitive man very lazy, and did he not do fewer things than he reasonably could have done? If we mean by lazy an aversion to certain types of action, primitive man was doubtless lazy; but if we mean an aversion to all kinds of exertion, he certainly was not lazy. He was so thoroughly aroused by certain stimulations and so exhausted by the expenditure of energy in reacting to these stimulations that periods of recuperation, or "sitting about," were necessary. Heckenwelder's remarks on the labor of men and women among the Indians of Pennsylvania are very instructive, although they relate to tribes which had come under white influences to some extent:

> The work of the women is not hard or difficult. They are both able and willing to do it, and always perform it with cheerfulness. Mothers teach their daughters those duties which common sense would otherwise point out to them when grown up. Within doors their labor is very trifling; there is seldom more than one pot or kettle to attend to. There is no scrubbing of the house, and but little to wash, and that not often. Their principal occupations are to cut and fetch in the firewood, till the ground, sow and reap the grain, and pound the corn in mortars for their pottage, and to make bread which they bake in the ashes. When going on a journey or to hunting camps with their husbands, if they have no horses, they carry a pack on their backs which often appears heavier than it really is; it generally consists of a blanket, a dressed deer skin for moccasins, a few articles of kitchen furniture, as a kettle, bowl, or dish, with spoons, and some bread, corn, salt, etc., for their nourishment. I have never known an Indian woman complain of the hardship of carrying this burden, which serves for their own comfort and support as well as of their husbands. The tilling of the ground at home, getting of firewood, and pounding of corn in mortars, is frequently done by female parties, much in the manner of those husking, quilting, and other *frolics* (as they are called) in some parts of

the United States.... [When accompanying her husband on the hunt the woman] takes pains to dry as much meat as she can, that none may be lost; she carefully puts the tallow up, assists in drying the skins, gathers as much wild hemp as possible for the purpose of making strings, carrying bands, bags, and other necessary articles; collects roots for dyeing; in short, does everything in her power to leave no care to her husband but the important one of providing meat for the family. After all, the fatigue of the women is by no means to be compared to that of the men. Their hard and difficult employments are periodical and of short duration, while their husbands' labors are constant and severe in the extreme. Were a man to take upon himself a part of his wife's duty, in addition to his own, he must necessarily sink under the load, and of course his family must suffer with him. On his exertions as a hunter their existence depends; in order to be able to follow that rough employment with success, he must keep his limbs as supple as he can, he must avoid hard labor as much as possible, that his joints may not become stiffened, and that he may preserve the necessary strength and agility of body to enable him to pursue the chase, and bear the unavoidable hardships attendant on it; for the fatigues of hunting wear out the body and constitution far more than manual labor. Neither creeks nor rivers, whether shallow or deep, frozen or free from ice, must be an obstacle to the hunter when in pursuit of a wounded deer, bear, or other animal, as is often the case. Nor has he then leisure to think on the state of his body, and to consider whether his blood is not too much heated to plunge without danger into the cold stream, since the game he is in pursuit of is running off from him with full speed. Many dangerous accidents often befall him both as a hunter and a warrior (for he is both), and are seldom unattended with painful consequences, such as rheumatism or consumption of the lungs, for which the sweat-house, on which they so much depend, and to which they often resort for relief, especially after a fatiguing hunt or warlike excursion, is not always a sure preservative or effectual remedy.[173]

The male and female come together by sexual attraction, and the chances of life are increased through association which permits each to do that class of things which by reason of its somatic habit it can do most effectively. Man's exploits were, however, of a more striking and sensational character, appealed to the emotions more, and secured the attention and the admiration of the public more, than the "drudgery" of the woman. The unusual esteem given by society to the destructive activities of the male can be very well understood in connection with a reference to the emotions. The emotions of anger, fear, and joy, to take only these examples, represent a physiological change in the organism in the presence of dangerous situations. Anger is a physiological preparation to resist, to crush a dangerous object; fear is an organic expression of inadequacy to avert the danger; and joy, in one of its aspects, is an organic revulsion answering to the recognition of the fact that the danger is safely passed. The same type of situation incessantly recurring in the life of the race, and constantly met by the same organic changes, has resulted in a fixed relation of certain types of situation to certain types of emotion.

The forms of activity recognized first of all in the consciousness of the race as virtuous are simply those which successfully avert danger and secure safety. Courage, intrepidity, endurance, skill, sagacity, an indomitable spirit, and a willingness to die in fight, are virtues of the first importance, vitally indispensable to the society in conflict with man and beast, and they are virtues of which man is by his organic constitution, by the very fact of his capacity for the rapid destruction of energy, particularly capable. Man's exploits, therefore, first of all had social attention.

The occupations of women were not of an emotional type, and, apart from sexual life, they got their excitements as spectators and approvers of the motor activities of the men. The Hebrew girls who went out with harps and timbrels to meet a victorious army, and sang that Saul had slain his thousands, but David his ten thousands, represent the relation between mighty deeds and social attention and approval. Thus the attention which the organism gives to situations of danger, through violent physiological readjustments fitted to meet the situation, has a parallel in the attention given by society to social means of meeting situations dangerous to the common life and welfare. We have a very plain continuance of the primitive appreciation of the virtues of violence in the worship of military men nowadays, and it is significant, also, that the appreciation of the fighting quality still reaches its most animated expression in women—the sex constitutionally most in need of social protection. It can hardly be denied, therefore, that man both enjoyed this exciting kind of performance more than the labors which women were connected with, and that the women justified him (if we assume that they passed any judgment on his conduct at all) in refraining from doing many things which he could have done perfectly well without constitutional hurt.

The abundance of the labors of primitive woman seems to be accounted for further by the fact that a stationary life is the condition of a greater variety of industrial expressions than a life inclined to motor expressions. It is notorious that a wandering life is not favorable to the development of industries. Industries, in their very nature, handle and shape stationary stuffs, for the most part, and woman developed the constructive or industrial activities as a simple consequence of her more stationary condition of life. The formation of habit is largely a matter of attention, and the attention of woman being limited by her bodily habit and the presence of children to objects lying closer at hand, her energies found expression in connection with these objects.

First of all, the house was identified with woman. The home was, in its simplest terms, the place where the wandering male rejoined the female. It was a cave, or a hollow tree, or a frail structure. It was sought or made with reference to safety and comfort, particularly with reference to the comfort of the young. Recognizing the greater interest of the woman in the child, it is evident that shelter was a more important consideration to her than to the man. The house is, indeed, a very fit accompaniment of the stationary habit of woman, and usually we find the most primitive tribes recognizing her greater interest in it. Even when the houses are built by men, they are generally owned by the women. Man as a solitary animal might, of course, make himself a shelter, but he had a particular interest in being about the shelter of woman, and it was under her shelter, after all, that children were born and that society accumulated numbers. This resulted in the maternal system and the recognition of woman as the head of the household, and the owner of the house. So, when the Indian squaw carries the wigwam on the march, she is carrying her private property and one of her own particular appurtenances. Contrary to the phrase which I quoted above, man is rather, in the sense in which I am now speaking, the domesticated animal. He has been inducted into the family. The estufas of the Pueblo Indians and the men's clubhouses in Africa represent the failure of men to assimilate completely in a society which was essentially female in its genius, and the club still stands for a difference in interest between the male and the female.

From the house, or shelter, as a base, woman got such connections with food as she might. For it is an error to suppose that she was in the most primitive times entirely dependent on man for food. She appears to have been quite as active in developing food surroundings in her way as man was in his. The plant world gave her the best returns for the effort which she could make. She beat out the seeds of plants, digged out the roots and tubers which the monkeys and pigs were seen to grub for most eagerly,[174] strained the poisonous juices from the cassava and made bread of the residue, and it was under her attention that a southern grass was developed into what we know as Indian corn. Looking back on this process, we call it the domestication of plants, and we are likely to regard it as a more conscious process than it really was. It was the result of her conversion to her own uses of the most available portion of her environment. In view of her physiological habit, the animal environment was, for the most part, out of the question, and her attention was of necessity directed to the plant side. While less remunerative in its beginnings than the animal side of the process, it was, perhaps, at all times less precarious and uncertain, and we find in consequence that the economic dependence of man on woman is as evident as her dependence on him. A dinner of herbs is a humbler resort than a roast of antelope, but there was less doubt that it would be forthcoming, and primitive man was often, when in hard luck, dependent on the activities of his wife, or the females of the group.

The domestication of animals appears similarly to be the following-up by man of his connections with animal life, when this life began to be less abundant. It is probable that the practice originated in the habit of taking the young of animals home as pets, and there is apparently a point of difference between the attention of the men and the women given to animals once taken into the household. The men were interested in these animals as reviving in memory the emotional situations of hunting life, and also in the clever and inimitable accuracy of co-ordination and superhuman development of sense-perceptions, while there was always in the attitude of woman toward these animals a touch of maternal feeling, such as is still expended on the "harmless, necessary cat." And, in a small way, woman also contributed to the domestication of animals by giving them suck, partly as an economic investment. In Tahiti and New Britain, for example, the women suckle the pigs, and the old women feed them.[175] Aside from this, the connections which primitive woman has with animal life is very slight. Worms and insects, shellfish, and even fish she may capture, but but after this her relation to animal life is in caring for the flesh and skins turned over to her by the man.

It was a very general early practice that, when man had killed his game and brought it home, he was not concerned in the further handling of it. He did not, indeed, in all cases bring it home, but sent his wife after it. The Indians killed buffalo only as fast as the squaws could cut them up and care for the meat, and the men of the Eskimos would not draw the seal from the water after spearing it. Exhausted by extraordinary efforts, the man may well have left the dressing of the animal upon occasion to his wife, and, exhausted or not, he soon fell into the habit of doing so. It thus turns out that all labors relating to the preparation of food, and to the utilizations of the side-products of food stuffs, are apt to be found in the hands of the women.

Vessels are necessary in cooking, both to carry and hold water, and to store the surplus of food, both vegetable and animal, and the woman, feeling the need of these in connection with what she has set about doing, weaves baskets and makes pottery. Fetching wood, grinding corn, tanning the hides, and in the main the preparation of clothing, follow rather necessarily from her relation to the raw products. Spinning and weaving and dyeing are related closely to the vegetable world to begin with, and it is to be expected that they would be developed by the women. But man is very deeply interested in clothing on the ornamental side, and the farther back we go in society, the more this holds, and sometimes, particularly in Africa, since the domestication of oxen there, the men prepare the leather and do the sewing, even for the women. There is, indeed, nothing in the nature of sewing to make it a woman's occupation. It involves a relation of the hand to the eye —similar to that which the man is always practicing and using, i.e., reaching a given point, perhaps with mechanical aids, through the mediation of these two organs. It is a motor matter, therefore, and one of the first industries undertaken by men. There are many exceptions to the general statement that early manufacture (weapons excepted) was in the hands of women, but the exceptions may be regarded as variations due to the fixation of habit through single and peculiar incidents, or they are the beginning of the later period when man begins to practice woman's activities.

The primitive division of labor among the sexes was not in any sense an arrangement dictated by the men, but a habit into which both men and women fell, to begin with, through their difference of organization—a socially useful habit whose rightness no one questioned and whose origin no one thought of looking into. There is, moreover, a tendency in habits to become more fixed than is inherently necessary. The man who does any woman's work is held in contempt not only by men, but by women.

> As to the Indian women, they are far from complaining of their lot. On the contrary, they would despise their husbands could they stoop to any menial office, and would think it conveyed an imputation upon their own conduct. It is the worst insult one virago can cast upon another in a moment of altercation. "Infamous woman," will she cry, "I have seen your husband carrying wood into the lodge to make the fire. Where was his squaw, that he should be obliged to make a woman of himself!"[176]

That men are similarly prejudiced against women's taking up male occupations we know from modern industrial history, without looking to ethnological evidence. Habit was, however, in another regard favorable to woman, since what she was constantly associated with and expended her activities upon was looked upon as hers. Through her identification with the industrial process she became, in fact, a property-owner. This result did not spring from the maternal system; but both this and the maternal system were the results of her bodily habit, and the social habits flowing from this.

> When the woman as cultivator was almost the sole creator of property in land, she held in respect of this also a position of advantage. In the transactions of North American tribes with the colonial governments

many deeds of assignments bear female signatures, which doubtless must also be referred to inheritance through the mother.[177]

Among the Spokanes "all household goods are considered as the wife's property."[178] The stores of roots and berries laid up by the Salish women for a time of scarcity "are looked upon as belonging to them personally, and their husbands will not touch them without having previously obtained their permission."[179] Among the Menomini a woman in good circumstances would possess as many as from 1,200 to 1,500 birch-bark vessels, and all of these would be in use during the season of sugar-making.[180] In the New Mexican pueblo,

> what comes from outside the house, as soon as it is inside is put under the immediate control of the woman. My host at Cochiti, New Mexico, could not sell an ear of corn or a string of *chile* without the consent of his thirteen-year-old daughter, Ignacia, who kept house for her widowed father. In Cholula district (and probably all over Mexico) the man has acquired more power, and the storehouse is no longer controlled by the wife. But the kitchen remains her domain; and its aboriginal designation, *tezcalli* (place, or house, of her who grinds), is still perfectly justified.[181]

> A plurality of wives is required by a good hunter, since in the labors of the chase women are of great service to their husbands. An Indian with one wife cannot amass property, as she is constantly occupied in household labors, and has not time for preparing skins for trading.[182]

The outcome of this closer attention of the woman to the industrial life is well seen among the ancient Hebrews:

> A virtuous woman ... seeketh wool and flax, and worketh willingly with her hands. She is like the merchant ships: she bringeth her food from afar. She riseth also while it is yet night, and giveth meat to her household, and their task to her maidens. She considereth a field and buyeth it; with the fruit of her hands she planteth a vineyard.... She perceiveth that her merchandise is profitable: her lamp goeth not out by night. She layeth her hands to the distaff, and her hands hold the

spindle. She spreadeth out her hand to the poor; yea, she reacheth forth her hands to the needy. She is not afraid of the snow for her household; for all her household are clothed with scarlet. She maketh for herself carpets of tapestry; her clothing is fine linen and purple. Her husband is known in the gates, when linen garments and selleth them; and delivereth girdles unto the merchant.[183]

There must come a time in the history of every group when wild game becomes scarce. This time is put off by successive migrations to wilder regions; but the rapid increase of population makes any continent inadequate to the supply of food through the chase indefinitely. Morgan estimates that the state of New York, with its 47,000 square miles, never contained at any one time more than 25,000 Indians.[184] Sooner or later the man must either fall back on the process represented by the women, taking up and developing her industries, or he must change his attitude toward animal life. In fact, he generally does both. He enters into a sort of alliance with animal life, or with certain of its forms, feeding them, and tending them, and breeding them; and he applies his katabolic energies to the pursuits of woman, organizing and advancing them. Whether the animal or the plant life receives in the end more attention is a matter turning on environment and other circumstances.

When the destructive male propensities have exhausted or diminished the food stores on the animal side, and man is forced to fall back on the constructive female process, we find that he brings greater and better organizing force to bear on the industries. Male enterprises have demanded concerted action. In order to surround a buffalo herd, or to make a successful assault, or even to row a large boat, organization and leadership are necessary. To attack under leaders, give signal cries, station sentinels, punish offenders, is, indeed, a part of the discipline even of animal groups. The organizing capacity developed by the male in human society in connection with violent ways of life is transferred to labor. The preparation of land for agriculture was undertaken by the men on a large scale. The jungle was cleared, water courses were diverted and highways prepared for the transportation of the products of labor.

But more than this, perhaps, man brought with him to the industrial occupations all the skill in fashioning force-appliances acquired through his intense, constant, and long-continued attention to the devising and manufacture of weapons. Man is relatively a feeble animal, but he made various and ingenious cutting, jabbing, and bruising appliances to compensate. His life was a life of strains, both giving and taking, and under the stress he had developed offensive and defensive weapons. There is, however, no radical difference, simply a difference in object and intensity of stimulus, between handling and making weapons and handling and making tools. So, when man was obliged to turn his attention to the agriculture and industries practiced by primitive woman he brought all his technological skill and a part of his technological interest to bear on the new problems. Women had been able to thrust a stick into the earth and drop the seed and await a meager harvest. When man turned his attention to this matter, his ingenuity eventually worked out a remarkable combination of the animal, mineral, and vegetable kingdoms: with the iron plow, drawn by the ox, he upturned the face of the earth, and produced food stuffs in excess of immediate demands, thus creating the conditions of culture.

The destructive habits of the male nature were thus converted under the stress of diminishing nutrition to the habits represented primarily by the constructive female nature, and the inventive faculty developed through attention to destructive mechanical aids was now applied equally to the invention of constructive mechanical aids.

SEX AND PRIMITIVE MORALITY

The function of morality is to regulate the activities of associated life so that all may have what we call fair play. It is impossible to think of morality aside from expressions of force, primarily physical force. "Thou shalt not kill; thou shalt not steal; thou shalt not bear false witness; thou shalt not commit adultery; thou shalt not remove the ancient landmark;" and all approvals and disapprovals imply that the act in question has affected or will affect the interest of others, or of society at large, for better or for worse. And since morality goes back so directly to forms of activity and their regulation, we may expect to find that the motor male and the more stationary female have had a different relation to the development of a moral code.

As between nutrition and reproduction, in the struggle for life, nutrition plays a larger rôle—in volume, at any rate—in the life-history of the individual. A consideration of the causes of the modification of species in nature shows that the changes in morphology and habit of the animal which relate to food-getting are more fundamental and numerous than those which relate to wooing. In a moral code, likewise, whether in an animal or human society, the bulk of morality turns upon food rather than sex relations; and since the male is more active in both these relations, and since, further, morality is the mode of regulating activities in these relations, it is to be expected that morality, and immorality as well, will be found primarily to a greater degree functions of the motor male disposition.

Tribal safety and the preservation and extension of the territory furnishing food demand the organized attention of the group first of all; and the emotional demonstrations and social rewards following modes of behavior which have a protective or provident meaning for the group, and the public disapproval and disallowance of modes of behavior which impair the safety or force capacity, and consequent satisfactions of the group, become in the tribe the most powerful of all stimuli, and stimuli to which the male is peculiarly able to react. This is not like the case of hunger and other physiological stimuli which are conditioned from within. The individual acts for the advantage of the group rather than for his personal advantage, and the stimulus to this action must be furnished socially. Group preservation being of first-rate importance, no group would survive in which the public showed apathy on this point. Lewis and Clarke say of the Dakota Indians:

> What struck us most was an institution peculiar to them and to the Kite Indians, further to the westward, from whom it is said to have been copied. It is an association of the most active and brave young men, who are bound to each other by attachment, secured by a vow never to retreat before any danger, or to give way to their enemies. In war they go forward without sheltering themselves behind trees, or aiding their natural valor by any artifice.... These young men sit, and encamp, and dance together, distinct from the rest of the nation; they are generally about thirty or thirty-five years old; and such is the deference paid to courage that their seats in the council are superior to those of the chiefs, and their persons more respected.[185]

The consciousness of the value of male activity is here expressed in an exaggerated degree—in a degree bordering upon the pathological, since the reckless exposure of life to danger is not necessary to success at a given moment, and is unjustifiable from the standpoint of public safety, unless it be on the side of the suggestive effect of intrepid conduct in creating a general standard of intrepidity. Similarly, the Indians in general often failed to get the full benefit of a victory, because of their practice that the scalp of an enemy belonged to him who took it, and their pursuits after a rout were checked by the delay of each to scalp his own.

The pedagogical attempts of primitive society, so far as they are applied to boys, have as an end the encouragement of morality of a motor, not a sentimental, type. The boys are taught war and the chase, and to despise the occupations of women. Thompson says of the Zulu boys:

> It is a melancholy fact that when they have arrived at a very early age, should their mothers attempt to chastise them, such is the law that these lads are at the moment allowed to kill their mothers.[186]

Ethnologists often make mention of the fact that the natural races do not generally punish children; and while this is due in part to a less definite sense of responsibility, as well as of less nervousness in parents, non-interference is a part of their system of training:

> Instead of teaching the boy civil manners, the father desires him to beat and pelt the strangers who come to the tent; to steal or secrete in joke some trifling article belonging to them; and the more saucy and impudent they are, the more troublesome to strangers and all the men of the encampment, the more they are praised as giving indication of a future enterprising and warlike disposition.[187]

Theft is also encouraged among boys as a developer of their wits. The Spartan boy and the fox is a classical example; and Diodorus relates that in Egypt the boy who wished to become a thief was required to enrol his name with the captain of the thieves, and to turn over to him all stolen articles. The citizens who were robbed went to the captain of thieves and recovered their property upon payment of one-fourth of its value.[188] Admiration of a lawless deed often foreruns censure of the deed in consciousness today: there are few men who do not admire a particularly daring and successful bank or diamond robbery, though they deprecate the social injury done.

Formally becoming a man is made so much of in early society, because it is on this occasion that fitness for activity is put to the test. Initiatory ceremonies fall at the time of puberty in the candidate, and consist of instruction and trials of fortitude. A certain show of the proceeds of activity is also exacted of young men, especially in connection with marriage, and the youth is not permitted to marry until he has killed certain animals or acquired certain trophies. The attention given to manly practices in connection with marriage is seen in this example from the Kukis:

> When a young man has fixed his affections upon a young woman, either of his own or some neighboring *Parah*, his father visits her father and demands her in marriage for his son: her father, on this, inquires what are the merits of the young man to entitle him to her favor; and how many can he afford to entertain at the wedding feast; to which the father of the young man replies that his son is a brave

warrior, a good hunter, and an expert thief; for that he can produce so many heads of the enemies he has slain and of the game he has killed; that in his house are such and such stolen goods; and that he can feast so many (mentioning the number) at his marriage.[189]

Occasionally the ability to take punishment is even made a part of the marriage ceremony. At Arab marriages

there is much feasting, and the unfortunate bridegroom undergoes the ordeal of whipping by the relations of his bride, in order to test his courage. Sometimes this punishment is exceedingly severe, being inflicted with the coorbatch, or whip of hippopotamus hide, which is cracked vigorously about his ribs and back. If the happy husband wishes to be considered a man worth having, he must receive the chastisement with an expression of enjoyment; in which case the crowds of women in admiration again raise their thrilling cry.[190]

A very simple record of successful activity is the bones of animals. McCosh says of the Mishmis of India:

Nor are these hospitable rites allowed to be forgotten; the skull of every animal that has graced the board is hung up as a record in the hall of the entertainer; he who has the best-stocked Golgotha is looked upon as the man of the greatest wealth and liberality, and when he dies the whole smoke-dried collection of many years is piled upon his grave as a monument of his riches and a memorial of his worth.[191]

And Grange of the Nagas:

In front of the houses of the greater folks are strung up the bones of the animals with which they have feasted the villagers, whether tigers, elephants, cows, hogs, or monkeys, or aught else, for it signifies little what comes to their net.[192]

The head-hunting mania of Borneo is also a pathological expression of the desire to get approval of destructive activity from both the living and the dead:

The aged of the people were no longer safe among their kindred, and corpses were secretly disinterred to increase the grizzly store. Superstition soon added its ready impulse to the general movement. The aged warrior could not rest in his grave till his relatives had taken a head in his name; the maiden disdained the weak-hearted suitor whose hand was not yet stained with some cowardly murder.[193]

Class distinctions and the attendant ceremonial observances go immediately back to an appreciation of successful motor activities. We need only observe the conduct of weaker animals in the presence of the stronger to appreciate the differences in behavior induced by the presence of superior motor ability. The recognition of this difference, as it is finally expressed in habitual forms of behavior, becomes a symbol of the difference, while the difference goes back, in reality, to a difference in capacity. This example from Raffles illustrates the intensity of moral meaning which the appreciation of achievement may take on in the end:

> At the court of *Súra-kérta* I recollect that once, when holding a private conference with the *Súsunan* at the residency, it became necessary for the *Rádan adipáti* to be dispatched to the palace for the royal seal: the poor old man was, as usual, squatting, and as the Susunan happened to be seated with his face toward the door, it was fully ten minutes before his minister, after repeated ineffectual attempts, could obtain the opportunity of rising sufficiently to reach the latch without being seen by his royal master. The mission on which he was dispatched was urgent, and the Susunan himself inconvenienced by the delay; but these inconveniences were insignificant compared with the indecorum of being seen out of the *dódok* posture. When it is necessary for an inferior to move, he must still retain that position, and walk with his hams upon his heels until he is out of his superior's sight.[194]

Drury says that a Malagasy chief, on his return from war,

> had scarcely seated himself at his door, when his wife came out crawling on her hands and knees until she came to him, and then licked his feet; when she had done, his mother did the same, and all the women in the town saluted their husbands in the same manner.[195]

An examination of the causes of the approval of conduct in early times thus discloses that approvals were based to a large degree on violent and socially advantageous conduct, that the training and rewards of early society were calculated to develop the skill and fortitude essential to such conduct, and that the men were particularly the representatives of conduct of this type. In the past, at any rate, there has been no glory like military glory, and no adulation like military adulation; and in the vulgar estimation still no quality in the individual ranks with the fighting quality.[196]

But checks upon conduct are even more definitely expressed, and more definitely expressible, than approvals of conduct. Approval is expressed in a more general expansive feeling toward the deserving individual, and this may be accompanied with medals for bravery, promotions, and other rewards; but in general the moral side of life gets no such definite notice as the immoral side. Practices which are disliked by all may be forbidden, while there is no equally summary way of dealing with practices approved by all. In consequence, practices which interfere with the activities of others are inhibited, and to the violation of the inhibition is attached a penalty, resulting in a body of law and a system of punishment. An analysis of the following crimes and punishments among the Kafirs, for instance, indicates that a definite relation between offensive forms of activity and punishments is present at a comparatively early period of development:

> Theft: restitution and fine. Injuring cattle: death or fine, according to the circumstances. Causing cattle to abort: heavy fine. Arson: fine. False witness: heavy fine. Maiming: fine. Adultery: fine, sometimes death. Rape: fine, sometimes death. Using love philters: death or fine, according to circumstances. Poisoning, and practices with an evil intent (termed "witchcraft"): death and confiscation. Murder: death or fine, according to circumstances.... Treason, as contriving the death of a chief, conveying information to the enemy: death and confiscation. Desertion from the tribe: death and confiscation.[197]

Similarly among the Kukis:

> Injuring the property of others, or taking it without payment; using violence; abusing parents; fraudulently injuring another; giving false

evidence; speaking disrespectfully to the aged; marrying an elder brother's wife; putting your foot on, or walking over, a man's body; speaking profanely of religion—are acts of impiety.[198]

As the vigorous and aggressive activities of the male have a very conspicuous value for the group when exercised for the benefit of the group, they become particularly harmful when directed against the safety or interests of the group or the members of the group, and we find that civil and criminal law, and contract, and also conventional morality, are closely connected with the motility of the male. The establishment of moral standards is mediated through the sense of strain—strain to the personal self, and strain to the social self. Whether a man is injured by an assault upon his life or upon his property, he suffers violence, and the first resort of the injured individual or group is to similar violence; but this results in a vicious tit-for-tat reaction whereby the stimulus to violence is reinstated by every fresh act of violence. Within the group this vicious action and reaction is broken up by the intervention of public opinion, either in an informal expression of disapproval, or through the headmen. The man who continues to kill may be killed in turn, but by order of the council of the tribe; and one of his kinsmen may be appointed to execute him, as under that condition no feud can follow. But there is always a reluctance to banish or take the life of the member of the group, both because no definite machinery is developed for accomplishing either, and because the loss of an able-bodied member of a group is a loss to the group itself. The group does not seek, therefore, immediately to be rid of an offensive member, but to modify his habits, to convert him. Jones says of the Ojibways that there were occasionally bad ones among them, "but the good council of the wise sachems and the mark of disgrace put upon unruly persons had a very desirable influence."[199] The extreme form of punishment in the power of the folk-moot of the Tuschinen is to be excluded from the public feasts, and to be made a spectator while stoned in effigy and cursed.[200] Sending a man to Coventry is in vogue among the Fejir Beduins: one who kills a friend is so despised that he is never spoken to again, nor allowed to sit in the tent of any member of the tribe.[201]

The formulation of sentiment about an act depends also on the repetition of the act. The act is more irritating, and the irritation more widespread, with each repetition, and there is an increase of the penalty for a second offense, and death for a slight offense when frequently repeated: in the Netherlands stealing of linen left in the fields to be bleached led to the death penalty for stealing a pocket handkerchief. And with increasing definiteness of authority there follows increasing definiteness of punishment; and when finally the habit becomes fixed, conformity with it becomes a paramount consideration, and a deed is no longer viewed with reference to its intrinsic import so much as to its conformity or nonconformity with a standard in the law: *summum jus, summa injuria*.

Morality, involving the modification of the conduct of the individual in view of the presence of others, is already highly developed in the tribal stage, since the exigencies of life have demanded the most rigorous regulation of behavior in order to secure the organization and the prowess essential to success against all comers. But the tribe is a unit in hostile coexistence with other similar units, and its morality stops within itself, and applies in no sense to strangers and outsiders. The North American Indians were theoretically at war with all with whom they had not concluded a treaty of peace. In Africa the traveler is safe and at an advantage if by a fiction (the rite of blood-brotherhood) he is made a member of the group; and similarly in Arabia and elsewhere. The old epics and histories are full of the praises of the man who is gentle within the group and furious without it. The earliest commandments doubtless did not originally apply to mankind at large. They meant, "Thou shalt not kill within the tribe," "Thou shalt not commit adultery within the tribe," etc. Cannibalism furnishes a most interesting example of the prohibition of a practice as applied to the members of the group, while extra-tribal cannibalism continued unabated. And within the tribe there is a continuance of this practice in the forms which do not interfere with the efficiency and cripple the activity of the group. That is, while cannibalism in general is prohibited, the eating of the decrepit, the aged, of invalids, of deformed children, and of malefactors is still practiced.[202]

But there gradually grew up a set of disapprovals of conduct as such, whether within or without the group. In the *Odyssey* Pallas Athene says that Odysseus had come from Ephyra from Ilus, son of Mermerus: "For even thither had Odysseus gone on his swift ship to seek a deadly drug, that he might have wherewithal to smear his bronze-shod arrows: but Ilus would in no wise give it to him, for he had in awe the everlasting gods."[203] Here is an extension to society in general of a principle which had been first worked out in the group; for poisoning without the group was long allowed after it was disallowed in the group. The case of poisoning is, indeed, a particularly good instance of an unsatisfaction felt in the substitution of clandestine methods for simple motor force in deciding a dispute, and affords a clear example of an important relation between moral feeling and physiological functioning. Animal as well as human society has developed strategy alongside of direct motor expressions, but strategy is only an indirect application of the motor principle. Co-ordination, associative memory, will, judgment, are involved in strategy; it is only a different mode of functioning. On the other hand, there is a peculiar abhorrence of murder by night, poisoning, drowning in a ship's hold, because, while all the physiological machinery for action is on hand, there is no chance to work it. It is a most exasperating thing to die without making a fight for it. The so-called American duel is an abhorrent thing, because life or death is decided by a turn of the dice, not on the racially developed principle of the battle to the strong.

When, then, it is observed within the group that this, that, and the other man has died of poison, each interprets this in terms of himself, and no one feels safe. The use of poison is not only a means of checking activities and doing hurt socially, but this form is most foul and unnatural because it involves a death without the possibility of motor resistance (except the inadequate opportunity on the strategic side of taking precautionary measures against poison) and a victory and social reward without a struggle. The group, therefore, early adopts very severe methods in this regard. Death is the usual penalty for the use of poison, and even the possession of poison, among tribes not employing it for poisoning weapons, is punished. Among the Karens of India, if a man is found with poison in his possession, he is bound and placed for three days in the hot sun, his poison is destroyed, and he is pledged not to obtain any more. If he is suspected of killing anyone, he is executed.[204] Particularly distressing modes of death, and other means of penalizing death by poison more severely than motor modes of killing, were adopted. The Chinese punish the preparation of poisons or capture of poisonous animals with beheading, confiscation, and banishment of wife and children. In Athens insanity caused by poison was punished with death. The *Sachsenspiegel* provides death by fire. In the lawbook of the tsar Wachtang a double composition price was exacted for death by poison. And in ancient Wales death and confiscation were the penalty for death by poison, and death or banishment the penalty of the manufacturer of poisons. The same quality of disapproval is expressed in early law of sorcery, and it is unnecessary to give details of this also. But, stated in emotional terms, both poison and sorcery, and other underhand practices arouse one of the most distressing of the emotions—the emotion of dread, if we understand by this term that form of fear which has no tangible or visible embodiment, which is apprehended but not located, and which in consequence cannot be resisted; the distress, in fact, lying in the inability to function. The organism which has developed structure and function through action is unsatisfied by an un-motor mode of decision. We thus detect in the love of fair play, in the Golden Rule, and in all moral practices a motor element; and with changing conditions there is progressively a tendency, mediated by natural selection and conscious choice, to select those modes of reaction in which the element of chance is as far as possible eliminated. This preference for functional over chance or quasi-chance forms of decision is expressed first within the group, but is slowly extended, along with increasing commercial communication, treaties of peace, and with supernatural assistance, to neighboring groups. The case of Odysseus is an instance of a moment in the life of the race when a disapproval is becoming of general application.

On our assumption that morality is dependent on strains, and that its development is due to the advantage of regulating these strains, we may readily understand why most of the canons of morality are functions of the katabolic male activity. Theft, arson, rape, murder, burglary, highway robbery, treason, and the like, are natural accompaniments of the more aggressive male disposition; the male is *par excellence* both the hero and the criminal. But on the side of the sex we might expect to find the female disposition setting the standards of morality, since reproduction is even a greater part of her nature than of man's. On the contrary, however, we find the male standpoint carried over and applied to the reproductive process, and the regulation of sex practices transpiring on the basis of force. In the earliest period of society, under the maternal system, the woman had her own will more with her person; but with the formulation of a system of control, based on male activities, the person of woman was made a point in the application of the male standpoint. "The wife, like any other of the husband's goods and chattels, might be sold or lent."[205] "Even when divorced she was by no means free, as the tribe exercised its jurisdiction in the woman's affairs and the disposal of her person."[206] Forsyth reports of the Gonds that

> infidelity in the married state is ... said to be very rare; and, when it does occur, is one of the few occasions when the stolid aborigine is roused to the extremity of passion, frequently revenging himself on the guilty pair by cutting off his wife's nose and knocking out the brains of her paramour with his ax.[207]

The sacrifice of wives in Africa, India, Fiji, Madagascar, and elsewhere, upon the death of husbands, shows how completely the person of the female had been made a part of the male activity. Where this practice obtained, the failure of the widow to acquiesce in the habit was highly immoral. Williams says of the strangling of widows by the Fijians:

> It has been said that most of the women thus destroyed are sacrificed at their own instance. There is truth in this statement, but unless other facts are taken into account it produces an untruthful impression. Many are importunate to be killed, because they know that life would henceforth be to them prolonged insult, neglect, and want.... If the friends of the woman are not the most clamorous for her death, their indifference is construed into disrespect either for her late husband or his friends.[208]

Child-marriages are another instance of the success of the male in gaining control of the person of the female and of regulating her conduct from his own standpoint. Girls were married or betrothed before birth, at birth, at two weeks, three months, or seven years of age, and variously, often to an adult, and their husbands were thus able to take extraordinary precautions against the violation of their chastity. On the other hand, it frequently happens, especially where marriage by purchase is not developed, that the conduct of the girl is not looked after until she is married; it becomes immoral only when disapproved by her husband. In the Andaman Islands, after puberty the females have indiscriminate intercourse ... until they are chosen or allotted as wives, when they are required to be faithful to their husbands, whom they serve.... If any married or single man goes to an unmarried woman, and she declines to have intercourse with him by getting up or going to another part of the circle, he considers himself insulted, and, unless restrained, would kill or wound her.[209]

Under these conditions the rightness or wrongness of the sexual conduct of the wife turned upon the attitude of the husband toward the act. Hence a very general practice that the husbands prostituted their wives for hire, but punished unapproved intercourse:

The chastity of the women does not appear to be held in much estimation. The husband will, for a trifling present, lend his wife to a stranger, and the loan may be protracted by increasing the value of the present. Yet, strange as it may seem, notwithstanding this facility, any connection of this kind not authorized by the husband is considered highly offensive and quite as disgraceful to his character as the same licentiousness in civilized societies.[210]

When woman lost the temporary prestige which she had acquired in the maternal system through her greater tendency to associated life, and particularly when her person came more absolutely into the control of man through the system of marriage by purchase, she also accepted and reflected naïvely the moral standards which were developed for the most part through male activities. Any system of checks and approvals in the group, indeed, which was of advantage to the men would be of advantage to the women also, since these checks and approvals were safeguards of the group as a whole, and not of the men only. The person and presence of woman in society have stimulated and modified male behavior and male moral standards, and she has been a faithful follower, even a stickler for the prevalent moral standards (the very tenacity of her adhesion is often a sign that she is an imitator); but up to date the nature of her activities—the nature, in short, of the strains she has been put to—has not enabled her to set up independently standards of behavior either like or unlike those developed through the peculiar male activities.

There is, indeed, a point of difference in the application of standards of morality to men and to women. Morality as applied to man has a larger element of the contractual, representing the adjustment of his activities to those of society at large, or more particularly to the activities of the male members of society; while the morality which we think of in connection with woman shows less of the contractual and more of the personal, representing her adjustment to men, more particularly the adjustment of her person to men.

THE PSYCHOLOGY OF EXOGAMY

Perhaps the most puzzling questions which meet the student of early society are connected with marriage and kinship; and among these questions the practice of exogamy has provoked a very large number of ingenious theories. These are, however, I believe, all unsatisfactory, either because they are too narrow to cover the facts completely, or because they assume in the situation conditions which do not exist.[211] But quite aside from the facts and the interpretation of the facts, all theories in the field have failed to reckon sufficiently with the natural disposition and habits of man in early society, particularly with his attitude toward sexual matters; and it seems entirely feasible to get some light on the question why man went outside his immediate family and clan for women through an examination of the nature of his sexual consciousness, and of the operation of this in connection with the laws of habit and attention.

First of all, it is evident to one who looks carefully into the question of early sex-habits that the lower races are intensely interested in sexual life. A large part of their thought, and even of their inventive ingenuity, is spent in this direction. The pleasures of life are few and gross, but are pursued with vigor; and, *mutatis mutandis*, love bears about the same relation to the activities of the Australian aborigine as it bore to those of Sir Lancelot and the knights of olden time.

A failure to perceive this is the great defect in Westermarck's great work, where it is assumed that, if animals were monogamous, primitive man must have been much the more so. The fact is that in respect to memory, imagination, clothing, mode of association, and social restraint man differed radically from the animals, and precisely through these added qualities he took not only an instinctive, but an artificial and reasoned, interest in sexual practices; and this resulted in a state of consciousness which made sexual life uninterruptedly interesting, in contrast with a pairing season among animals, and also in a constant tendency toward promiscuity, whether this state was ever actually reached or not. The widespread and various unnatural sex practices, the use of aphrodisiacs, the practice of drawing attention to the girl at puberty, phallic worship, erotic dances, and periodic orgies, of which the Orient furnishes so many examples, are all found also among the natural races.[212]

Again, the eagerness of men to obtain girl wives, and even a claim on infants, thus assuring virginity and marriage at the moment of sexual maturity;[213] the habit of keeping girls in solitary confinement from a tender age until the consummation of marriage;[214] and the African custom of infibulation,[215] are classes of facts indicating that the sexual element occupied a large place in the consciousness of the natural races.

We must also consider the fact that sexual life is organically a utilization of a surplus of nutriment, and that when food and leisure are abundant there is a tendency on the part of sexual activity to become a play activity, just as there is a tendency of activities in general to become play activities under the same conditions. And while there was no leisure class in early society, primitive man was a man of leisure in the sense that his work activities were intermittent; a successful hunt was followed by a period of rest, recuperation, and surplus energy, and a consequent turning of attention to sexual life, with the result that the sex interest appears as one of the main play interests among the natural races.

Under these conditions, and in the absence of any considerably developed social institutions or altruistic sentiments, we not unnaturally find that the older and stronger men have the better of it, both in regard to the food supply and the women, and the younger men are obstructed in their efforts to satisfy their desires in regard to both. The following passages from the ethnological literature of Australia indicate the nature of the Australian male in sexual life, and the nature of the obstructions encountered by the youth in the presence of the older men.[216]

It is noticeable, first of all, that among the Australian tribes the older men have worked out or fallen into such habits regarding the females that the younger men obtain wives with great difficulty and usually not before waiting a long time. In fact, Spencer and Gillen, in their invaluable works on the central Australian tribes state that usually a man is married to a woman of another generation than himself:

The most usual method of obtaining a wife is that which is connected with the well-established custom in accordance with which every woman of the tribe is made *Tualcha mura* with some man. The arrangement, which is often a mutual one, is made between two men, and it will be seen that owing to a girl being made *Tualcha mura* to a boy of her own age the men very frequently have wives much younger than themselves, as the husband and the mother of the wife obtained in this way are usually approximately of the same age. When it has been agreed upon by two men that the relationship shall be established between their own children, one a boy and the other a girl, the two latter, who are generally of a tender age, are taken to the *Erlukwirra*, or women's camp, and here each mother takes the other child and rubs it over with a mixture of fat and red ochre.... This relationship indicates that the man has the right to take as wife the daughter of the woman; she is in fact assigned to him, and this, as a rule, many years before she is born.[217]

It will be noticed that this is in reality a modification of the system of exchanging women, and has an advantage over capture, elopement, and charming (all of which are methods in practice among the same tribes) in the fact that it is of the nature of a business transaction or social agreement, and provokes no bad feeling or retaliation. It also shows considerable regard on the part of the elders for the young; but practically it is a reluctant admission of a youth to participation in sexual privileges, since marriage is delayed until a girl of his own age has been married and given birth to a girl who in turn has become marriageable.

In the same connection we have the testimony of Curr that

the marriage customs of the blacks result in very ill-assorted unions as regards age; for it is usual to see old men with mere girls as wives, and men in the prime of life married to old widows. As a rule wives are not obtained by the men until they are at least thirty years of age. Women have very frequently two husbands during their lifetime, the first older and the second younger than themselves. Of course, as polygamy is the rule and the men of the tribe exceed the females in number besides, there are always many bachelors in every tribe; but I never heard of a female over sixteen years of age who, prior to the breakdown of aboriginal customs after the coming of the whites, had not a husband.[218]

And Bonwick says:

The old men, who get the best food and hold the franchise of the tribe in their hands, manage to secure an extra supply of the prettiest girls.[219]

A further evidence of the keen sexual interest of the male is furnished by the fact that even when the difficulties in the way of getting a wife are regularly overcome by the youth, the other men of the group, especially the older ones, reserve a temporary but prior claim on her.[220]

In addition to a lively sexual interest in the women of their own group, we find that even the lowest races have a well-developed appreciation of the property value of women. In the earliest times women were the sole creators of certain economic values, and since the women contributed as much or more to the support of the men as the men contributed to the support of the women, the men naturally got and kept as many women as possible.[221] The condition prevailing in this regard in central Australia is stated by Howitt:

It is an advantage to a man to have as many *Piraurus* as possible. He has then less work to do in hunting as his *Piraurus* when present supply him with a share of the food which they procure, their own *Noas* being absent. He also obtains great influence in the tribe by lending his *Piraurus* occasionally and receiving presents from young men to whom *Piraurus* have not yet been allotted, or who may not have *Piraurus* with them in the camp where they are. This is at all times carried on, and such a man accumulates a lot of property, weapons of all kinds, trinkets, etc., which he in turn gives away to prominent men, heads of totems, and such, and thus adds to his own influence. This is regarded by the Dieri as in no way anything but quite right and proper.[222]

The following passages also from Spencer and Gillen's description of the marriage customs of these aborigines show both the nature of the sexual system of these tribes in general and the well-developed nature of both their sexual and their property interest in their women:

The word *Nupa* is without any exception applied indiscriminately by men of a particular group to women of another group, and *vice versa*, and simply implies a member of a group of possible wives or husbands, as the case may be. While this is so it must be remembered that in actual practice each individual man has one or perhaps two of these *Nupa* women who are especially attached to himself, and live with him in his own camp. In addition to them, however, each man has certain *Nupa* women beyond the limited number just referred to, with whom he stands in the relation of *Piraungaru*. To women who are the *Piraungaru* of a man (the term is a reciprocal one) the latter has access under certain conditions, so that they may be considered as accessory wives. The result is that in the Urabunna tribe every woman is the especial *Nupa* of one particular man, but at the same time he has no exclusive right to her as she is the *Piraungaru* of certain other men who also have the right of access to her. Looked at from the point of view of the man his *Piraungaru* are a limited number of the women who stand in the relation of *Nupa* to him. There is no such thing as one man having the exclusive right to one woman; the elder brothers, or *Nuthie*, of the latter, in whose hands the matter lies, will give one man a preferential right, but at the same time they will give other men of the same group a secondary right to her. Individual marriage does not exist either in name or in practice in the Urabunna tribe. The initiation in regard to establishing the relationship of *Piraungaru* between a man and a woman must be taken by the elder brothers, but the arrangement must receive the sanction of the old men of the group before it can take effect. As a matter of actual practice this relationship is usually established at times when considerable numbers of the tribe are gathered together to perform important ceremonies, and when these and other important matters which require the consideration of the old men are discussed and settled. The number of a man's *Piraungaru* depends entirely upon the measure of his power and popularity; if he be what is called "urku," a word which implies much the same as our word "influential," he will have a considerable number; if he be insignificant or unpopular, then he will meet with scanty treatment. A woman may be *Piraungaru* to a number of men, and as a general rule the women and men who are *Piraungaru* to one another are to be found living grouped together. A man may always lend his wife, that is, the woman to whom he has the first right, to another man, provided always he be her *Nupa*, without the relationship of *Piraungaru* existing between the two, but unless this relationship exists no man has any right of access to a woman. Occasionally, but rarely, it happens that a man attempts to prevent his wife's *Piraungaru* from having access to her, but this leads to a fight, and the husband is looked upon as churlish.[223]

The evidence up to this point is presented with a view to establishing the fact that the men in early society had the strongest interest, both on sexual and on property grounds, in retaining a hold on the women of their group; and as an extreme expression of this interest I wish to consider the system of elopement in early society. While there is no system of government by chiefs among the Australian tribes which we have been considering, the influence of the old men is very powerful in all matters. The initiatory ceremonies, covering periods of months and occurring at intervals during a period of years, and involving great hardship to the young men, are calculated to inspire them with great respect for the old men and for the traditional practices of the tribe. One of the practical workings of this influence of the older men is to throw restraints about the young men and obstruct their activities. This obstruction is seen quite as clearly on the food side as on the side of sex, in the fact that the old men make certain foods which are not abundant (notably the kangaroo and the opossum) taboo to the young men and the women, and thus reserve these delicacies for themselves. We have already seen, however, that the tribe usually makes some kind of a tardy sexual provision for its male members, and we shall presently examine this question more in detail; but the fact remains that the desires of the young men are not adequately or promptly provided for. They may never get a wife in the usual course of things, or they may have to delay marriage for a period of twenty years beyond the point of maturity. Under these conditions it is to be expected that the young men should sometimes attempt to obtain women in spite of existing obstructions; and this is the real significance of elopement. It is, of course, true that married men sometimes eloped with married women, as with us; but in some of the Australian tribes the difficulties in the way of marriage were so great that elopement was recognized as the only way out:

> The young Kurnai could, as a rule, acquire a wife in one way only. He must run away with her. Native marriage might be brought about in various ways. If the young man was so fortunate as to have an unmarried sister and to have a friend who also had an unmarried sister they might arrange with the girls to run off together or he might make his arrangements with some eligible girl whom he fancied and who fancied him; or a girl, if she fancied some young man might send him a secret message asking, "Will you find me some food?" and this was understood to be a proposal. But in every case it was essential for success that the parents of the bride should be utterly ignorant of what was about to transpire.[224]

Fison[225] is of the opinion that elopement in this case is caused by the monopoly of women in the tribe by the older men. Even when the assent of the parents has been secured, or when the match has been arranged by the parents of the young people, it is in some cases necessary to elope because of the reluctance of the men in general to have a young woman appropriated:

> If the woman was caught her female relatives gave her a good beating. Fights took place over these cases between the girl's relatives—both male and female—and those of the man. The women were generally the most excited; they would stir up the men and then assist with their yamsticks. If the girl was first caught by other than her own relatives, she would be abused by all the men; but this never occurred when her parents or brothers were present to protect her.[226]

When we consider the difficulties in the way of young men in getting wives at home, we should expect that they would make a practice of capturing women from other tribes; and, indeed, it is well known that marriage by capture has been assumed to be at the base of exogamy by both Lubbock and Spencer. But the importance which has been attached to this form of marriage in the literature of sociology is due to the fact that these eminent writers have constructed theories on the assumption that marriage by capture was widespread and important, more than to anything else. For, to say nothing of the fact that the theories of both these writers are too weak to stand even if capture were found to be very prevalent, the evidence from Australia shows that capture was comparatively little practiced there, although that country affords most of the examples referred to by writers on this subject. Spencer and Gillen say in this connection:

> The method of capture which has so frequently been described as characteristic of Australian tribes, is the very rarest way in which the Central Australian secures a wife. It does not often happen that a man forcibly takes a woman from someone else within his own group, but it does sometimes happen, and especially when the man from whom the woman is taken has not shown his respect for his actual or tribal *Ikuntera* (father-in-law) by cutting himself on the occasion of the death of one or the other of the latter's relations. In this case the aggressor will be aided by the members of his local group, but in other cases of capture he will have to fight for himself. At times, however, a woman may be captured from another group, though this again is of rare occurrence, and is usually associated with an avenging party, the women captured by which, who are almost sure to be the wives of men killed, are allotted to certain members of the avenging party.[227]

Curr reports to the same effect:

> On rare occasions a wife is captured from a neighboring tribe and carried off.... At present, as the stealing of a woman from a neighboring tribe would involve the whole tribe in war for his sole benefit, and as the possession of the woman would lead to constant attacks, tribes set themselves generally against the practice.[228]

It is, of course, not to be denied that the sexual impulse of the male was sometimes strong enough to lead him to seize a woman wherever he found her, if he could not get a wife otherwise, but there is no evidence that capture ever formed a regular or important means of getting wives.[229]

On the contrary, the evidence points to the view that as soon as for any reason men ceased to marry with the women of their own blood and went outside of their immediate families for women, they ordinarily secured them in a social, not a hostile, way, and from a different branch of their own group, not, as a rule, from a strange group. In fact, the regular means of securing a wife other than a woman of one's own family seems to have been to exchange a woman of one's family for a woman of a different family.

The Australian male almost invariably obtains his wife or wives either as the survivor of a married brother, or in exchange for his sisters, or later on in life for his daughters. Occasionally also an ancient widow, whom the rightful heir does not claim, is taken possession of by some bachelor but for the most part those who have no female relatives to give in exchange have to go without wives. Girls become wives at from eight to fourteen years. Males are free to possess wives after ... attaining the status of young man, which they do when about eighteen years of age. One often sees a child of eight the wife of a man of fifty. Females until married are the property of their father or his heir, and afterwards of their husband, and have scarcely any rights. When a man dies his widows devolve on his oldest surviving brother of the same caste as himself—that is, full brother. Should a man leave, say two widows, each of whom has a son who has attained the rank of a young man, then I believe each of the young men may dispose of his uterine sister and obtain a wife in exchange for her. But should the deceased father of the young men have already obtained wives on faith of giving these daughters in marriage when of suitable age, then the contract made must be kept. When the father is old and his sons young men, it happens sometimes that he barters females at his disposal for wives for them.[230]

Roth also reports[231] that exchange of sisters is one mode of negotiating marriage; and Haddon says that in the region of Torres Straits marriage is proposed by the woman, but the man must either pay for her or furnish a woman in return. In Tud, after the young people have come to an agreement, they both go home and tell their respective relatives. "For girl more big (i.e., of more consequence) than boy." If the girl has a brother, he takes the man's sister, and then all is settled. The fighting does not appear to be a very serious business.[232]

Similarly in Maibung:

An exchange of presents and foods was made between the contracting parties, but the bridegroom's friends had to give the larger amount, and the bridegroom had to pay the parents for his wife, the usual price being a canoe or dugong harpoon, or shell armlet, or goods to equal value. The man might give his sister in exchange for a wife, and thus save the purchase price. A poor man who had no sister might perforce remain unmarried, unless an uncle took pity on him and gave him a cousin to exchange for a wife.[233]

Fison and Howitt[234] give other examples of marriage by exchange, and I have already given a description of the custom of *Tualcha mura*, the *regular* method of obtaining a wife among the central Australians, by means of which a man secures a wife for his son by making an arrangement with some other man with regard to the latter's daughter.

From the evidence given first of all I think we must conclude that early man was inclined to appropriate whatever women came in his way. In this regard we have a condition resembling that among the higher animals, where the more vigorous males try to monopolize the females. We may assume also that the women first appropriated were those born in the group—that is, in the immediate family—as being more proximate and not already possessed by others. In this regard also the condition resembled that among the higher gregarious animals; and in so far as the control of the women by the men of the group is concerned the condition remains unchanged. But the men have ceased to marry the women of their immediate families, and the problem of exogamy is to determine why men living with women and controlling them should cease to marry them.

In other papers I have pointed out that the interest of man is not held nor the emotions aroused when the objects of attention have grown so familiar in consciousness that the problematical and elusive elements disappear;[235] and I have also alluded to the laws of sexual life, that an excited condition of the nervous system is a necessary preparation to pairing.[236] And just here we must recognize the fact that monogamy is a habit acquired by the race, not because it has answered more completely to the organic interest of the individual, but because it has more completely served social needs, particularly by assuring to the woman and her children the undivided interest and providence of the man. But in early times the law of natural selection, not the law of choice, operated to preserve the groups in which a monogamous or quasi-monogamous tendency showed itself (since the children in these cases were better trained and nourished), and in historical times and among ourselves all of the machinery of church and state has been set in motion in favor of the system. In point of fact, the members of civilized societies at the present time have become so refined and have so far accepted ethical standards that monogamy is the system actually favored on sentimental grounds as well as on grounds of expediency by a large proportion of any civilized population. On the other hand, speaking from the biological standpoint, monogamy does not, as a rule, answer to the conditions of highest stimulation, since here the problematical and elusive elements disappear to some extent, and the object of attention has grown so familiar in consciousnes that the emotional reactions are qualified. This is the fundamental explanation of the fact that married men and women frequently become interested in others than their partners in matrimony. I may also just allude to the fact that the large body of the literature of intrigue, represented by the tales of Boccaccio and Margaret of Navarre, is based on the interest in unfamiliar women.

Familiarity with women within the group and unfamiliarity with women without the group is the explanation of exogamy on the side of interest; and the system of exogamy is a result of exchanging familiar women for others. We have seen that capture was not an important means of securing wives outside the group, and that exogamy was fully developed before property and media of exchange were developed to any extent, and consequently before the purchase of women had become a system. We have seen also that the Australian who wants a woman at the present time gets her by exchanging another woman for her. Social groups were necessarily small in the beginning. Before invention and co-operation have advanced far, the group must remain small in order to pick up enough food to sustain life on a given area.

Starting out with a single pair, when the family increases in size a separation is necessary; and clans are an outcome of the process of division and redivision, the bond between the clans and their union in a tribe resulting from their consciousness of kinship. Now, it is a well-known condition of exogamy that, while a man must marry without his clan, he must not marry without his tribe, and for the most part, in fact, the clan into which he shall marry is designated. In other words, allied clans gave their women in exchange mutually. This was a natural arrangement, both because the two groups were neighbors and because they were friendly, and at the same time the psychological demand for newness was satisfied. When a family was divided into two branches, Branch A had a property interest in its own women, but preferred the women of Branch B because of their unfamiliarity. The exchange took place at first occasionally and not systematically, and the women parted with in each case were not, perhaps, in all cases the youngest, and we may assume that they had in all cases been married before they were given up. But gradually, and when the habit of exchange had been established, men came to look forward to the exchange and to desire to secure the girl at the earliest possible moment, until finally young women were exchanged at puberty, and virgins. When for any reason there is established in a group a tendency toward a practice, then the tendency is likely to become established as a habit, and regarded as right, binding, and inevitable: it is moral and its contrary is immoral. When we consider the binding nature of the food taboos, of the *couvade*, and of the regulation that a man shall not speak to or look at his mother-in-law or sister, we can understand how the habit of marrying out, introduced through the charm of unfamiliarity, becomes a binding habit.

I think, therefore, we have every reason to conclude that exogamy is one expression of the more restless and energetic habit of the male. It is psychologically true that only the unfamiliar and not-completely-controlled is interesting. This is the secret of the interest of modern scientific pursuit and of games. States of high emotional tension are due to the presentation of the unfamiliar—that is, the unanalyzed, the uncontrolled—to the attention. And although the intimate association and daily familiarity of family life produce affection, they are not favorable to the genesis of romantic love. Cognition is so complete that no place is left for emotional appreciation. Our common expressions "falling in love" and "love at sight" imply, in fact, unfamiliarity; and there can be no question that men and women would prefer at present to get mates away from home, even if there were no traditional prejudice against the marriage of near kin.

THE PSYCHOLOGY OF MODESTY AND CLOTHING

No altogether satisfactory theory of the origin of modesty has been advanced. The naïve assumption that men were ashamed because they were naked, and clothed themselves to hide their nakedness, is not tenable in face of the large mass of evidence that many of the natural races are naked, and not ashamed of their nakedness; and a much stronger case can be made out for the contrary view, that clothing was first worn as a mode of attraction, and modesty then attached to the act of removing the clothing; but this view in turn does not explain an equally large number of cases of modesty among races which wear no clothing at all. A third theory of modesty, the disgust theory, stated by Professor James[237] and developed somewhat by Havelock Ellis,[238] makes modesty the outgrowth of our disapproval of immodesty in others—"the application in the second instance to ourselves of judgments primarily passed upon our mates."[239] The sight of offensive behavior is no doubt a powerful deterrent from like behavior, but this seems to be a secondary manifestation in the case of modesty. The genesis of modesty is rather to be found in the activity in the midst of which it appears, and not in the inhibition of activity like the activity of others. It appears also that it has primarily no connection with clothing whatever.[240]

Professor Angell and Miss Thompson have made an investigation of the relation of circulation and respiration to attention, which advances considerably our knowledge of the nature of the emotions. They say:

> When the active process runs smoothly and uninterruptedly, these bodily activities [circulation and respiration] progress with rhythmic regularity. Relatively tense, strained attention is generally characterized by more vigorous bodily accompaniments than is low-level, gentle, and relatively relaxed attention (drowsiness, for instance); but both agree, so long as their progress is free and unimpeded, in relative regularity of bodily functions. Breaks, shocks, and mal-co-ordinations of attention are accompanied by sudden,

spasmodic changes and irregularities in bodily processes, the amount and violence of such changes being roughly proportioned to the intensity of the experiences.

Now, emotions represent psychological conditions of great instability. Especially is this true when the emotion is profound. The necessity is suddenly thrown upon the organism of reacting to a situation with which it is at the moment able to cope only imperfectly, if at all. The condition is one in which normal, uninterrupted, coordinated movements are for a time checked and thrown out of gear.[241]

And again, in concluding their admirable study:

All the processes with which we have been dealing are cases of readjustment of an organism to its environment. Attention is always occupied with the point in consciousness at which the readjustment is taking place. If the process of readjustment goes smoothly and evenly, we have a steady strain of attention—an equilibrated motion in one direction. The performance of mental calculation is a typical case of this sort of attention. But often the readjustment is more difficult. Factors are introduced which at first refuse to be reconciled with the rest of the conscious content. The attentive equilibrium is upset, and there are violent shifts back and forth as it seeks to recover itself. These are the cases of violent emotion. Between these two extremes comes every shade of difficulty in the readjustment, and of consequent intensity in emotional tone. We have attempted to show in the preceding paper that the readjustment of organism to environment involves a maintenance of the equilibrium of the bodily processes, which runs parallel with the maintenance of the attentive equilibrium, and is an essential part of the readjustment of the psycho-physical organism.

The more motile organisms are constantly, by very reason of their motility, encountering situations which put a strain upon the attention. The quest for food leads to encounters with members of their own and of different species; the resulting fight, pursuit, and flight are accompanied by the powerful emotions of anger and fear. The emotion is, as Darwin has pointed out, a part of the effort to reaccommodate, since it is a physiological preparation for action appropriate to the type of situation in question.[242] The strain upon the attention, the affective bodily condition, and the motor activity appear usually in the same connection, and, from the standpoint of biological design, the action concluding the series of bodily activities is of advantage to the organism.

In animal life the situation is simple. Whether the animal decides to fight for it or to run for it, he has at any rate two plain courses before him, and the relation between his emotional states and the type of situation is rather definitely fixed racially, and relatively constant. Even in the associated life of animals the type of reaction is not much changed, and is here also instinctively fixed. But in mankind the instinctive life is overshadowed or rivaled by the freedom of initiative secured through an extraordinary development of the power of inhibition and of associative memory, while, at the same time, this freedom of choice is hindered and checked by the presence of others. The social life of mankind brings out a thousand situations unprovided for in the instincts and unanticipated in consciousness. In the midst, then, of a situation relatively new in race experience, where advantage is still the all-important consideration, and where this can no longer be secured either by fighting or running, but by the good opinion of one's fellows as well, we may look for some new strains upon the attention and some emotions not common to animal life.

I do not think we can entirely understand the nature of these emotional expressions in the race unless we realize that man is, in his savage as well as his civilized state, enormously sensitive to the opinion of others.[243] The longing of the Creek youth to "bring in hair" and be counted a man; the passion of the Dyak of Borneo for heads, and the recklessness of the modern soldier, "seeking the bubble reputation at the cannon's mouth;" the alleged action of the young women of Kansas in taking a vow to marry no man who had not been to the Philippine war, and of the ladies of Havana, during the rebellion against Spain, in sending a chemise to a young man who stayed at home, with the suggestion that he wear it until he went to the field—all indicate that the opinion of one's fellows is at least as powerful a stimulus as any found in nature. To the student of ethnology no point in the character of primitive man is more interesting and surprising than his vanity. This unique susceptibility to social influence is, indeed, essential to the complex institutional and associational life of mankind. The transmission of language, tradition, morality, knowledge, and all race experience from the older to the younger, and from one generation to another, is accomplished through mental suggestibility, and the activity of the individual in associational life is mediated largely through it.

Now, taking them as we find them, we know that such emotions as modesty and shame are associated with actions which injure and shock others, and show us off in a bad light. They are violations of modes of behavior which have become habitual in one way and another. In an earlier paper[244] have indicated some of the steps by which approvals and disapprovals were set up in the group. When once a habit is fixed, interference with its smooth running causes an emotion. The nature of the habit broken is of no importance. If it were habitual for *grandes dames* to go barefoot on our boulevards or to wear sleeveless dresses at high noon, the contrary would be embarrassing. Psychologically the important point is that, when the habit is set up, the attention is in equilibrium. When inadvertently or under a sufficiently powerful stimulus we break through a habit, the attention and associative memory are brought into play. We are conscious of a break, of what others will think; we anticipate a damaged or diminished personality; we are, in a word, upset. We may consequently expect to find that whatever brings the individual into conflict with the ordinary standards of life of the society in which he is living is the occasion of a strain on the attention and of an accompanying bodily change.[245]

A minimum expression of modesty, and one having an organic rather than a social basis, is seen in the coyness of the female among animals. In many species of animals the female does not submit at once to the solicitations of the male, but only after the most arduous wooing.

> The female cuckoo answers the call of her mate with an alluring laugh that excites him to the utmost, but it is long before she gives herself up to him. A mad chase through tree tops ensues, during which she constantly incites him with that mocking call, till the poor fellow is fairly driven crazy. The female kingfisher often torments her devoted lover for half a day, coming and calling him, and then taking to flight. But she never lets him out of her sight the while, looking back as she

flies, and measuring her speed, and wheeling back when he suddenly gives up the pursuit.[246]

There is here a rapid shifting of attention between organic impulse to pair and organic dread of pairing, until an equilibrium is reached, which is not essentially different from the case, in human society, of that woman who, "whispering, 'I will ne'er consent,' consented." In either case, the minimum that it is necessary to assume is an organic hesitancy, though in the case of woman social hesitancy may play even the greater rôle. Pairing is in its nature a seizure, and the coquetry of the female goes back, perhaps, to an instinctive aversion to being seized.

Our understanding of the nature of modesty is here further assisted by the consideration that the same stimulus does not produce the same reaction under all circumstances, but, on the contrary, may result in totally contrary effects. A show of fight may produce either anger or fear; social attention may gratify us from one person and irritate us from another; or the attentions of the same person may annoy us today and please us tomorrow. Mere movement is, to take another instance, one of the most powerful stimuli in animal life; and, if we examine its meaning among animals, we find that the same movement may have different meanings in terms of sex. If the female runs, the movement attracts the notice of the male, and the movement is a sexual stimulus. Or the movement may be a movement of avoidance—a running-away; and in this way the female may secure contrary desires by the same general type of activity. Or, on the other hand, not-running is a condition of pairing, and is also a means of avoiding the attention of the male. Similarly modesty has a twofold meaning in sexual life. In appearance it is an avoidance of sexual attention, and at many moments it is an avoidance in fact. But we have seen in the case of the birds that the avoidance is, at the pairing season, only a part of the process of working up the organism to the nervous pitch necessary for pairing.

But without going farther into the question of the psychology of wooing, it is evident that very delicate attention to behavior is necessary to be always attractive and never disgusting to the opposite sex, and even the most serious attention to this problem is not always successful.[247] Sexual association is a treacherous ground, because our likes and dislikes turn upon temperamental traits rather than on the judgment, or, at any rate, upon modes of judgment not clearly analyzable in consciousness. An openness of manner in the relations of the sexes is very charming, but a little more, and it is boldness, or, if it relates to bodily habits, indecency. A modest behavior is charming, but too much modesty is prudery. Under these circumstances, when the suggestive effect of bodily habits is realized, but the effect of a given bit of behavior cannot be clearly reckoned, and when, at the same time, the effect produced by the action is felt to be very important to happiness, it is to be expected that there should often be a conflict between the tendency to follow a stimulus and the tendency to inhibit it, a hovering between advance and retreat, assent and negation—a disturbed state of attention, and an organic hesitancy, resulting in the emotional overflow of blushing when the act is realized or thought as improper.

But, however thin and movable the partitions between attraction and disgust, every person is aware of certain standards of behavior, derived either from the strain of personal relationship or by imitation of current modes of behavior. The girl of the unclothed races who takes in sitting a modest attitude is acting on the result of experience. She may have been often annoyed by the attentions of men at periods when their attention was not welcome, and in this case the action is one of shrinking and avoidance. She doubtless has in mind also that all females are not at all times attractive to all males, that female boldness sometimes excites disgust, and that the concealment of the person may be more attractive than its exposure.

This more or less instinctive recognition of the suggestive power of her person and her corresponding attitude of modesty have been assisted also by her observation of the experiences of other women, and by the talk of the older women. I may add the following instances to make it plain that the sexual relation is the object of much attention from both sexes in primitive society, and furnishes occasion for the interruption of the smooth flow of the attention and the bodily activities. Describing the use of magic by the male Australians in obtaining wives, Spencer and Gillen add:

> In the case of charming, however, the initiative may be taken by the woman, who can, of course, imagine that she has been charmed, and then find a willing aider and abettor in the man, whose vanity is

flattered by the response to the magic power which he can soon persuade himself that he did really exercise.[248]

If this attempt at suggestion failed, we should have a case of lively embarrassment in the woman, and her discomfiture would be heightened if the other women and men of the community were aware of her attempt. Similarly on Jervis Island in Torres Straits, if an unmarried woman was interested in a man, she accosted him, but the man did not address the woman "for, if she refused him, he would feel ashamed, and maybe he would brain her with a stone club, and so 'he would kill her for nothing.'"[249]

A wholesale unsettling of habit is seen when a lower culture is impinged upon by a higher. The consciousness of other standards of behavior causes new forms of modesty in the lower race. Haddon reports of the natives of Torres Straits:

> The men were formerly nude, and the women wore only a leaf petticoat, but I gather that they were a decent people; now both sexes are prudish. A man would never go nude before me—only once or twice has it happened to me, and then only when they were diving.... Amongst themselves they are, of course, much less particular, but I believe they are becoming more so.... I have not noticed any reticence in their speaking about sexual matters before the young, but missionary influence has modified this a great deal; formerly, I imagine, there was no restraint in speech, now there is a great deal of prudery;... and I had the greatest possible difficulty in getting the little information I did about the former relationships between the sexes. All this, I suspect, is not really due to a sense of decency *per se*, but rather to a desire on their part not to appear barbaric to strangers; in other words, the hesitancy is between them and the white man, not as between themselves.[250]

Bonwick says also:

> I have repeatedly been amused at observing the Australian natives prepare for their approach to the abode of civilization by wrapping

their blankets more decently around them and putting on their ragged trousers or petticoats.[251]

There are numerous cases found among the lower races where the wearing of clothing and ornament are not associated with feelings of modesty. Von den Steinen reports that the women of Brazil wore a small, delicately made and ornamented covering or *uluri*, which evidently had an attractive as well as protective value; but the women showed no embarrassment, but rather astonishment, when he asked them to remove them and give them to him. When they understood that he really wanted them, they removed them and gave them to him with a laugh.[252] This is a case, in fact, of the beginning of clothing without a beginning of modesty. But while we find cases of modesty without clothing and of clothing without modesty the two are usually found together, because clothing and ornament are the most effective means of drawing the attention to the person, sometimes by concealing it and sometimes by emphasizing it.

The original covering of the body was in the nature of ornament rather than clothing. The waist, the neck, the wrists, and the ankles are smaller than the portion of the body immediately below them, and are from this anatomical accident a suitable place to tie ornaments, and the ornamentation of the body results incidently in giving some degree of covering to the body. The most suggestive use of clothing is the use of just a sufficient amount to call attention to the person, without completely concealing it. I need not refer to the fact that in modern society this is accomplished by, or perhaps we should better say transpires in connection with, diaphanous fabrics and décolleté dresses; and the same effect was doubtless accomplished by a typical early form of female dress, of which I will give one instance in Australia and one in America:

Among the Arunta and Luricha the women normally wear nothing, but amongst tribes farther north, especially the Kaitish and Warramunga, a small apron is made and worn, and this sometimes finds its way south into the Arunta. Close-set strands of fur-string hang vertically from a string waist-girdle. Each strand is about eight or ten inches in length, and the breadth of the apron may reach the same size, though it is often not more than six inches wide.[253]

Mr. Powers says:

> A fashionable young Wittun woman wears a girdle of deer skin, the lower edge of which is slit into a long fringe, with the polished pine-nut at the end of each strand, while the upper border and other portions are studded with brilliant bits of shell.[254]

If we recall the psychological standpoint that the emotions are an organic disturbance of equilibrium occurring when factors difficult of reconciliation are brought to the attention, and if we have in mind that the association of the sexes has furnished so powerful an emotional disturbance as jealousy, it seems a simple matter to explain the comparatively mild by-play of sexual modesty as a function of wooing, without bringing either clothing or ornament into the question.

We saw a minimum expression of modesty in the courtship of animals, where the modesty of the female was a form of fear on the organic side, but the accompanying movements of avoidance were, at the same time, a powerful attraction to the male. And we have in this, as in all expressions of fear—shame, guilt, timidity, bashfulness—an affective bodily state growing out of the strain thrown upon the attention in the effort of the organism to accommodate itself to its environment. The essential nature of the reaction is already fixed in types of animal life where the operation of disgust is out of the question, and in relations which imply no attention to the conduct of others. If any separation between the bodily self and the environment is to be made at all, it is putting the cart before the horse to make out that modesty is derived from our repugnance at the conduct of others, more immediately than through attention to the meaning of our own activities. The fallacy of the disgust theory lies, in fact, in the attempt to separate the copies for imitation derived from our own activities from those derived from our observation of the activities of others.

When habits are set up and are running smoothly, the attention is withdrawn; and nakedness was a habit in the unclothed societies, just as it may become a habit now in the artist's model. But when, for any of the reasons I have outlined, women or men began to cover the body, then putting off the covering became peculiarly suggestive, because the breaking-up of a habit brings an act clearly into attention. And when dress becomes habitual in a society whose sense of modesty has also developed to a high degree, the suggestive effect is so great that the bare thought of unclothing the person becomes painful, and we have the possibility of such a phenomenon as mock modesty. But, so far as sexual modesty is concerned, the clothing has only reinforced the already great suggestive power of the sexual characters.

In animal society the coyness of the female is the analogue of modesty. The male is always aggressive, and in both animal and human society used ornament as a means of interesting and influencing the female. In the course of time, however, man's activities became his main dependence, and woman's person and personal behavior became more significant, especially in a state of society where she became dependent on man's activities, and both ornament and modesty were largely transferred to her.

In speaking of the relation of sex to morality,[255] I have already shown that the morality of man is peculiarly a morality of prowess and contract, while woman's morality is to a greater degree a morality of bodily habits, both because child-bearing, which is a large factor in determining sexual morality, is more closely connected with her person, and in consequence also of male jealousy. Physiologically and socially reproduction is more identified with the person of woman than of man, and it has come about that her sexual behavior has been more closely looked after, not only by men, but by women—for it would not be difficult to show that women have been always, as they are still, peculiarly watchful of one another in this respect.

In the course of history woman developed an excessive and scrupulous concern for the propriety of her behavior, especially in connection with her bodily habits; and this in turn became fixed and particularized by fashion, with the result that not only her physical life became circumscribed, but her attention and mental interests became limited largely to safeguarding and enhancing her person.

The effect of this and of other similar restrictions of behavior on her character and mind is indicated in following chapters.

THE ADVENTITIOUS CHARACTER OF WOMAN

There is more than one bit of evidence that nature changed her plan with reference to some organism at the very last moment, and introduced a feature which was not contemplated at the outset. This change of plan is carried out through the specialization of some organ, sense, or habit, to such a degree as to make practically a new type of the organism. In the human species, for example, the atrophied organs distributed through the body are evidence that the physical make-up of the species was well-nigh definitely fixed before the advantage of free hands led to an erect posture, thereby throwing certain sets of muscles out of use; and the specialization of the voice as a means of communicating thought was, similarly, a device for relieving the hands of the burden of communication, and was not introduced systematically until a gesture language had been so well established that even now we fall back into it unconsciously, especially in moments of excitement, and attempt to talk with our hands and bodies.

But perhaps the most interesting modification or reversal of plan to be noted in mankind is connected with the relation of the two sexes. As will presently be indicated, life itself was in the beginning female, so far as sex could be postulated of it at all, and the life-process was primarily a female process, assisted by the male. In humankind as well, nature obviously started out on the plan of having woman the dominant force, with man as an aid; but after a certain time there was a reversal of plan, and man became dominant, and woman dropped back into a somewhat unstable and adventitious relation to the social process. Up to a certain point, in fact, in his physical and social evolution man shows an interesting structural and mental adaptation to woman, or to the reproductive process which she represents; while the later stages of history show, on the other hand, that the mental attitude of woman, and consequently her forms of behavior, have been profoundly modified, and even her physical life deeply affected, by her effort to adjust to man.

The only attitude which nature can be said to show toward life is the design that the individual shall sustain its own life, and at death leave others of its kind—that it shall get food, avoid destruction, and reproduce. In pursuance of this policy it naturally turns out that those types showing greater morphological and functional complexity, along with freer movement and more mental ingenuity, come into the more perfect control and use of their environment, and consequently have greater likelihood of survival. Failing of this greater complexity, their chance of life lies in occupying so obscure a position, so to speak, that they do not come into collision with more dominant forms, or in reproducing at such a rate as to survive in spite of this. The number of devices in the way of modification of form and habit to secure advantage is practically infinite, but all progressive species have utilized the principle of sex as an accessory of success. By this principle greater variability is secured, and among the larger number of variations there is always a chance of the appearance of one of superior fitness. The male in many of the lower forms is very insignificant in size, economically useless (as among the bees), often a parasite on the female, and, as many biologists hold, merely a secondary device or afterthought of nature, designed to secure greater variation than can be had by the asexual mode of reproduction. In other words, he is of use to the species by assisting the female to reproduce progressively fitter forms.

When, in the course of time, sexual reproduction eventuated in a mammalian type, with greater intimacy between mother and offspring and a longer period of dependence of offspring on the mother, the function of the male in assisting the female became social as well as biological; and this was pre-eminently so in the case of man, because of the pre-eminent helplessness of the human child.[256] The characteristic helplessness of the child, which at first thought appears to be a disadvantage, is in fact the source of human superiority, since the design of nature in providing this condition of helplessness is to afford a lapse of time sufficient for the growth of the very complex mechanism, the human brain, which, along with free hands, is the medium through which man begins that reaction on his environment—inventing, exterminating, cultivating, domesticating, organizing—which ends in his supremacy.

It is plain, therefore, that species in which growth is slow are at an advantage, if to the care and nourishment of the female are added the providence and protection of the male; and this is especially true in mankind, where growth is not completed for a long period of years. In this connection we have an explanation of the alleged greater variability of the male. Instead of an insignificant addendum to the reproductive process, he becomes larger than the female, masterful, jealous, a fighting specialization —still an attaché of the female, but now a defender and provider. This is the general condition among mammals; and among mankind the longer dependence of children results in a correspondingly lengthened and intimate association of the parents, which we denominate marriage. For Westermarck is quite right in his view that children are not the result of marriage, but marriage is the result of children. From this point of view marriage is a union favored by the scheme of nature because it is favorable to the rearing and training of children, and the groups practicing marriage, or its animal analogue, have the best chance of survival.

But the evolution of a courageous and offensive disposition naturally did not result in an eminently domestic disposition. Man did the hunting and fighting. He was attached to the woman, but he was not steady. He did not stay at home. The woman and the child were the core of society, the fixed point, the point to which man came back. There consequently grew up a sort of dual society and dual activity. Man represented the more violent and spasmodic activities, involving motion and skillful co-ordinations, as well as organization for hunting and fighting; while woman carried on the steady, settled life. She was not able to wander readily from a fixed point, on account of her children; and, indeed, her physical organization fitted her for endurance rather than movement. Consequently her attention was turned to industries, since these were compatible with settled and stationary habits. Agriculture, pottery, weaving, tanning, and all the industrial processes involved in working up the by-products of the chase, were developed by her. She domesticated man and assisted him in domesticating the animals. She built her house, and it was hers. She did not go to her husband's group after marriage. The child was hers, and remained a member of her group. The germ of social organization was, indeed, the woman and her children and her children's children. The old women were the heads of civil society, though the men had developed a fighting organization and technique which eventually swallowed them up.

From the standpoint of physical force, man was the master, and was often brutal enough. But woman led an independent life, to some extent. She was, if not economically independent, at least economically creative, and she enjoyed the great advantage of being less definitely interested in man than he was in her. For while woman is more deeply involved physiologically in the reproductive life than man, she is apparently less involved from the standpoint of immediate stimulus, or her interest is less acute in consciousness. The excess activity which characterizes man in his relation to the general environment holds also for his attitude toward woman. Not only is the male the wooer among the higher orders of animals and among men, but he has developed all the accessories for attracting attention—in the animals, plumage, color, voice, and graceful and surprising forms of motion; and in man, ornament and courageous action. For primitive man, like the male animal, was distinguished by ornament.

Up to this time the relation of man to woman was the natural development of a relation calculated to secure the best results for the species. His predacious disposition had been, in part at least, developed in the service of woman and her child, and he was emotionally dependent on her to such a degree that he used all the arts of attraction at his command to secure a relation with her. In the course of time, however, an important change took place in environmental conditions. While woman had been doing the general work and had developed the beginnings of many industries, man had become a specialist along another line. His occupation had been almost exclusively the pursuit of animals or conflict with his neighbors; and in this connection he had become the inventor of weapons and traps, and in addition had learned the value of acting in concert with his companions. But a hunting life cannot last forever; and when large game began to be exhausted, man found himself forced to abandon his destructive and predacious activities, and adopt the settled occupations of woman. To these he brought all the inventive technique and capacity for organized action which he had developed in his hunting and fighting life, with the result that he became the master of woman in a new sense. Not suddenly, but in the course of time, he usurped her primacy in the industrial pursuits, and through his organization of industry and the application of invention to the industrial processes became a creator of wealth on a scale before unknown. Gradually also he began to rely not altogether on ornament, exploits, and trophies to get the attention and favor of woman. When she was reduced to a condition of dependence on his activity, wooing became a less formidable matter; he purchased her from her male kindred, and took her to his own group, where she was easier to control.

In unadvanced stages of society, where machinery and the division of labor and a high degree of organization in industry have not been introduced, and among even our own lower classes, woman still retains a relation to industrial activities and has a relatively independent status. Among the Indians of this country it was recognized that a man could not become wealthy except through the possession of a sufficient number of wives to work up for trade the products of the chase; and today the West African youth does not seek a young woman in marriage but an old one, preferably a widow, who knows all about the arts of preparing and adulterating rubber. Among peasants, also, and plain people the proverb recognizes that the "gray mare is the better horse." The heavy, strong, enduring, patient, often dominant type, frequently seen among the lower classes, where alone woman is still economically functional, is probably a good representative of what the women of our race were before they were reduced by man to a condition of parasitism which, in our middle and so-called higher classes, has profoundly affected their physical, mental, and moral life.

On the moral side, particularly, man's disposition to bend the situation to his pleasure placed woman in a hard position and resulted in the distortion of her nature, or rather in bringing to the front elemental traits which under our moral code are not reckoned the best. In the animal world the female is noted for her indirection. On account of the necessity of protecting her young, she is cautious and cunning, and, in contrast with the open and pugnacious methods of the more untrammeled male, she relies on sober colors, concealment, evasion, and deception of the senses. This quality of cunning is, of course, not immoral in its origin, being merely a protective instinct developed along with maternal feeling. In woman, also, this tendency to prevail by passive means rather than by assault is natural; and especially under a system of male control, where self-realization is secured either through the manipulation of man or not at all, a resort to trickery, indirection, and hypocrisy is not to be wondered at. Man has, however, always insisted that woman shall be better than he is, and her immoralities are usually not such as he greatly disapproves. There has, in fact, been developed a peculiar code of morals to cover the peculiar case of woman. This may be called a morality of the person and of the bodily habits, as contrasted with the commercial and public morality of man. Purity, constancy, reserve, and devotion are the qualities In woman which please and flatter the jealous male; and woman has responded to these demands both really and seemingly. Without any consciousness of what she was doing (for all moral traditions fall in the general psychological region of habit), she acts in the manner which makes her most pleasing to men. And —always with the rather definite realization before her of what a dreadful thing it is to be an old maid—she has naïvely insisted that her sisters shall play well within the game, and has become herself the most strict censor of that morality which has become traditionally associated with woman. Fearing the obloquy which the world attaches to a bad woman, she throws the first stone at any woman who bids for the favor of men by overstepping the modesty of nature. Morality, in the most general sense, represents the code under which activities are best carried on, and is worked out in the school of experience. It is pre-eminently an adult and a male system, and men are intelligent enough to recognize that neither women nor children have passed through this school. It is on this account that, while man is merciless to woman from the standpoint of personal behavior, he exempts her from anything in the way of contractual morality, or views her defections in this regard with allowance and even with amusement.

In the absence of any participation in commercial activity and with no capital but her personal charms and her wits, and with the possibility of realizing on these only through a successful appeal to man, woman naturally puts her best foot first. It was, of course, always one of the functions of the female to charm the male; but so long as woman maintained her position of economic usefulness and her quasi-independence she had no great problem, for there was never a chance in primitive society, any more than in animal society, that a woman would go unmated. But when through man's economic and social organization, and the male initiative, she became dependent, and when in consequence he began to pick and choose with a degree of fastidiousness, and when the less charming women were not married—especially when "invidious distinctions" arose between the wed and unwed, and the desirably wed and the undesirably wed-woman had to charm for her life; and she not only employed the passive arts innate with her sex, but flashed forth in all the glitter which had been one of man's accessories in courtship, but which he had dispensed with when the superiority acquired through occupational pursuits enabled him to do so. Under a new stimulation to be attractive, and with the addition of ornament to the repertory of her charms, woman has assumed an almost aggressive attitude toward courtship. The means of attraction she employs are so highly elaborated, and her technique is so finished, that she is really more active in courtship than man. We speak of man as the wooer, but falling in love is really mediated by the woman. By dress, behavior, coquetry, modesty, reserve, and occasional boldness she gains the attention of man and infatuates him. He does the courting, but she controls the process. "Er glaubt zu schieben, und er wird geschoben."

The condition of limited stimulation, also, in which woman finds herself as a result of the control by man of wealth, of affairs, of the substantial interests of society, and even of her own personality, leads woman to devote herself to display as an interest in itself, regardless of its effect on men. In doing this she is really falling back on an instinct. One of the most powerful stimulations to either sex is glitter, in the most general sense, and the interest in showing off begins in the coloration and plumage of animals, and continues as ornament in the human species. It is true that the wooing connotation of ornament was originally its most important one, and that it was characteristic of man in particular; but woman has generalized it as an interest, and as a means of self-realization. She seeks it as a means of charming men, of outdoing other women, and as an artistic interest; and her attention often takes that direction to such a degree that its acquisition means satisfaction, and its lack discontent. Sometimes, indeed, when a woman is married and knows that she is "sped," she drops the display pose altogether, tends to lose herself in household interests, and to become a slattern. On the other hand, she often makes marriage the occasion of display on a more elaborate scale, and is pitiless in her demands for the means to this. A glance at the windows of our great stores shows that men have organized their business in a full appreciation of these facts. Dressing, indeed, becomes a competitive game with women, and since their opponents and severest critics are women, it turns out curiously enough that they dress even more with reference to the opinion of women than for men.

The earth hath bubbles as the water has,
And these are of them.

It would, of course, be absurd to censure woman too greatly for these frailties, and it would be very unjust to imply that all women share them. Some women, in adapting themselves to the situation, follow apparently, a bent acquired in connection with the maternal instinct, and become true and devoted and grand to a degree hardly known by man. Others, following a bent gotten along with coquetry in connection with the wooing instinct, and having no activity through which their behavior is standardized, become difficile, unreal, inefficient, exacting, unsatisfied, absurd. And we have also the paradox that the same woman can be the two things at different times. There is therefore a basis of truth in Pope's hard saying that "Women have no characters at all." Because their problem is not to accommodate to the solid realities of the world of experience and sense, but to adjust themselves to the personality of men, it is not surprising that they should assume protean shapes.

Moreover, man is so affected by the charms of woman, and offers so easy a mark for her machinations, as to invite exploitation. Having been evolved largely through the stimulus of the female presence, he continues to be more profoundly affected by her presence and behavior than by any other stimulus whatever, unless it be the various forms of combat. From Samson and Odysseus down, history and story recognize the ease and frequency with which a woman makes a fool of a man. The male protective and sentimental attitude is indeed incompatible with resistance. To charm, pursue, court, and possess the female, involve a train of memories which color all after-relations with the whole sex. In both animals and men there is an instinctive disposition to take a great deal off the female. The male animal takes the assaults of the female complacently and shamefacedly, "just like folks." Peasants laugh at the hysterical outbreaks of their women, and the "bold, bad man" is as likely to be henpecked as any other. Woman is a disturbing element in business and in school to a degree not usually apprehended. In her presence a man instinctively assumes a different attitude. He is, in fact, so susceptible as seemingly, almost, to want to be victimized, and, as Locke expressed the matter, "It is in vain to find fault with those arts of deceiving wherein men find pleasure to be deceived."

This disposition of man and the detached condition of woman have much to do with the emergence of the adventuress and the sporting-woman. Human nature was made for action; and perhaps the most distressing and disconcerting situation which confronts it is to be played on by stimulations without the ability to function. The mere superinducing of passivity, as in the extreme case of solitary confinement, is sufficient to produce insanity; and the emotion of dread, or passive fear, is said to be the most painful of emotions, because there is no possibility of relief by action. Modern woman is in a similar condition of constraint and unrest, which produces organic ravages for which no luxury can compensate. The general ill-health of girls of the better classes, and the equally general post-matrimonial breakdown, are probably due largely to the fact that the nervous organization demands more normal stimulations and reactions than are supplied. The American woman of the better classes has superior rights and no duties, and yet she is worrying herself to death—not over specific troubles, but because she has lost her connection with reality. Many women, more intelligent and energetic than their husbands and brothers, have no more serious occupations than to play the house-cat, with or without ornament. It is a wonder that more of them do not lose their minds; and that more of them do not break with the system entirely is due solely to the inhibitive effects of early habit and suggestion.

As long as woman is comfortably cared for by the men of her group or by marriage, she is not likely to do anything rash, especially if the moral standards in her family and community are severe. But an unattached woman has a tendency to become an adventuress—not so much on economic as on psychological grounds. Life is rarely so hard that a young woman cannot earn her bread; but she cannot always live and have the stimulations she craves. As long, however, as she remains with her people and is known to the whole community, she realizes that any infraction of the habits of the group, any immodesty or immorality, will ruin her standing and her chance of marriage, and bring her into shame and confusion.

Consequently, good behavior is a protective measure—instinctive, of course; for it is not true that the ordinary girl has imagination enough to think out a general attitude toward life other than that which is habitual in her group. But when she becomes detached from home and group, and is removed not only from surveillance, but from the ordinary stimulation and interest afforded by social life and acquaintanceship, her inhibitions are likely to be relaxed.

The girl coming from the country to the city affords one of the clearest cases of detachment. Assuming that she comes to the city to earn her living, her work is not only irksome, but so unremunerative that she finds it impossible to obtain those accessories to her personality in the way of finery which would be sufficient to hold her attention and satisfy her if they were to be had in plenty. She is lost from the sight of everyone whose opinion has any meaning for her, while the separation from her home community renders her condition peculiarly flat and lonely; and she is prepared to accept any opportunity for stimulation offered her, unless she has been morally standardized before leaving home. To be completely lost sight of may, indeed, become an object under these circumstances—the only means by which she can without confusion accept unapproved stimulations—and to pass from a regular to an irregular life and back again before the fact has been noted is not an unusual course.

The professionally irregular class of women represents an extreme and unfortunate result of an adventitious and not-completely-functional relation to society. They do not form a class in the psychological sense, but only a trade. There are many sorts of natural dispositions among them—as many perhaps as will be found in any other occupation. None of the reputable occupations are homogeneous from the standpoint of the natural dispositions of the men and women who compose them, and the same is true of the disreputable occupations. Many women of fine natural character and disposition are drawn in a momentary and incidental way into an irregular life, and recover, settle down to regular modes of living, drift farther, are married, and make uncommonly good wives. In this respect the adventuress is more fortunate than the criminal (that other great adventitious product), because the criminal is labeled and his record follows him, making reformation difficult; while the in-and-out life of woman with reference to what we call virtue is not officially noted and does not bring consequences so inevitable. But "if you drive nature out at the door, she will come back through the window;" and this interest in greater stimulation is, I believe, the dominant force in determining the choice—or, rather, the drift —of the so-called sporting-woman. She is seeking what, from the psychological standpoint, may be called a normal life.

The human mind was formed and fixed once for all in very early times, through a life of action and emergency, when the species was fighting, contriving, and inventing its way up from the sub-human condition; and the ground-patterns of interest have never been, and probably never will be, fundamentally changed. Consequently, all pursuits are irksome unless they are able, so to speak, to assume the guise of this early conflict for life in connection with which interest and modes of attention were developed. As a matter of fact, however, anything in the nature of a problem or a pursuit stimulates the emotional centers, and is interesting, because it is of the same general pattern as these primitive pursuits and problems. Scientific and artistic pursuits, business, and the various occupational callings are analogues of the hunting, flight, pursuit, courtship, and capture of early racial life, and the problems they present may, and do, become all-absorbing. The moral and educational problem of development has been, indeed, to substitute for the simple, co-ordinative killing, escaping, charming, deceiving activities of early life, analogues which are increasingly serviceable to society, and to expand into a general social feeling the affection developed first in connection with courtship, the rearing of children, and joint predatory and defensive enterprises. The gamester, adventuress, and criminal are not usually abnormal in a biological sense, but have failed, through defective manipulation of their attention, to get interested in the right kind of problems. Their attention has not been diverted from interests of a primary type containing a maximum of the sensory, to interests of an analogous type containing more elements of reflection, and involving problems and processes of greater benefit to society.

The remedy for the irregularity, pettiness, ill-health, and unserviceableness of modern woman seems to lie, therefore, along educational lines. Not in a general and cultural education alone, but in a special and occupational interest and practice for women, married and unmarried. This should be preferably gainful, though not onerous nor incessant. It should, in fact, be a play-interest, in the sense that the interest of every artist and craftsman, who loves his work and functions through it, is a play-interest. Normal life without normal stimulation is not possible, and the stimulations answering to the nature of the nervous organization seem best supplied by interesting forms of work. This reinstates racially developed stimulations better than anything except play; and interesting work is, psychologically speaking, play.

Some kind of practical activity for women would also relieve the strain on the matrimonial situation—a situation which at present is abnormal and almost impossible. The demands for attention from husbands on the part of wives are greater than is compatible with the absorbing general activities of the latter, and women are not only neglected by the husband in a manner which did not happen in the case of the lover, but they are jealous of men in a more general sense than men are jealous of women. In the absence of other interests they are so dependent on the personal interest that they unconsciously put a jealous construction, not only on personal behavior, but on the most general and indifferent actions of the men with whom their lives are bound up; and this process is so obscure in consciousness that it is usually impossible to determine what the matter really is.

An examination, also, of so-called happy marriages shows very generally that they do not, except for the common interest of children, rest on the true comradeship of like minds, but represent an equilibrium reached through an extension of the maternal interest of the woman to the man, whereby she looks after his personal needs as she does after those of the children—cherishing him, in fact, as a child—or in an extension to woman on the part of the man of that nurture and affection which is in his nature to give to pets and all helpless (and preferably dumb) creatures.

Obviously a more solid basis of association is necessary than either of these two instinctively based compromises; and the practice of an occupational activity of her own choosing by woman, and a generous attitude toward this on the part of man, would contribute to relieve the strain and to make marriage more frequently successful.

THE MIND OF WOMAN AND THE LOWER RACES

I

The mind is a very wonderful thing, but it is questionable whether it is more wonderful than some of the instinctive modes of behavior of lower forms of life. If mind is viewed as an adjustment to external conditions for the purpose of securing control, the human mind is no more wonderful in its way than the homing and migratory instincts of birds; the tropic quality of the male butterfly which leads it to the female though she is imprisoned in a cigar-box in a dark room; or the peculiar sensitivity of the bat which enables it, though blinded, to thread its way through a maze of obstructions hung about a room.

The fact of sensitivity, in short, or the quality of response to stimulation, is more wonderful than its particular formulation in the human brain. Mind simply represents a special development of the quality of sensitivity common to organic nature, and analogous to the sensitivity of the photographic plate. The brain receives impressions, records them, remembers them, compares new experiences with old, and modifies behavior, in the presence of a new or recurrent stimulation, in view of the pleasure-pain connotation of similar situations in the past.

In very low forms of life, as is well known, there is no development of brain or special organs of sense; but the organism is pushed and pulled about by light, heat, gravity, and acid and other chemical forces, and is unable to decline to act on any stimulus reaching it. It reacts in certain characteristic, habitual, and adequate ways, because it responds uniformly to the same stimulation; but it has no choice, and is controlled by the environment. The object of brain development is to reverse these conditions and control the actions of the organism, and of the outside world as well, from within. With the development of the special organs of sense, memory, and consequent ability to compare present experiences with past, with inhibition or the ability to decline to act on a stimulus, and, finally, with abstraction or the power of separating general from particular aspects, we have a condition where the organism sits still, as it were, and picks and chooses its reactions to the outer world; and, by working in certain lines to the exclusion of others, it gains in its turn control of the environment, and begins to reshape it.

All the higher animals possess in some degree the powers of memory, judgment, and choice; but in man nature followed the plan of developing enormously the memory, on which depend abstraction, or the power of general ideas, and the reason. In order to secure this result, the brain, or surface for recording experience, was developed out of all proportion with the body. In the average European the brain weighs about 1,360 grams, or 3 per cent. of the body weight, while the average brain weight of some of the great anthropoid apes is only about 360 grams, or, in the orangoutang, one-half of 1 per cent. of the body weight. In point of fact, nature seems to have reached the limit of her materials in creating the human species. The development of hands freed from locomotion and a brain out of proportion to bodily weight are *tours de force*, and, so to speak, an afterthought, which put the heaviest strain possible on the materials employed, and even diverted some organs from their original design. A number of ailments like hernia, appendicitis, and uterine displacement, are due to the fact that the erect posture assumed when the hands were diverted from locomotion to prehensile uses put a strain not originally contemplated on certain tissues and organs. Similarly, the proportion of idiocy and insanity in the human species shows that nature had reached the limit of elasticity in her materials and began to take great risks. The brain is a delicate and elaborate organ on the structural side, and in these cases it is not put together properly, or it gets hopelessly out of order. This strain on the materials is evident in all races and in both sexes, and indicates that the same general structural ground-pattern has been followed in all members of the species.

Viewed from the standpoint of brain weight, all races are, broadly speaking, in the same class. For while the relatively small series of brains from the black race examined by anthropologists shows a slight inferiority in weight —about 45 grams in negroes—when compared with white brains, the yellow race shows more than a corresponding superiority to the white; in the Chinese about 70 grams. There is also apparently no superiority in brain weight in modern over ancient times. The cranial capacity of Europeans between the eleventh and eighteenth centuries, as shown by the cemeteries of Paris, is not appreciably different from that of Frenchmen of today, and the Egyptian mummies show larger cranial capacity than the modern Egyptians. Furthermore, the limits of variation between individuals in the same race are wider than the average difference between races. In a series of 500 white brains, the lowest and highest brains will differ, in fact, as much as 650 grams in weight.

There is also no ground for the assumption that the brain of woman is inferior to that of man; for, while the average brain of woman is smaller, the average body weight is also smaller, and it is open to question whether the average brain weight of woman is smaller in proportion to body weight.[257] The importance of brain weight in relation to intelligence, moreover, has usually been much exaggerated by anthropologists; for intelligence depends on the rapidity and range of the acts of associative memory, and this in turn on the complexity of the neural processes. Brains are, in fact, like timepieces in this respect, that the small ones work "excellent well" if they are good material and well put together. Although brains occasionally run above 2,000 grams in weight (that of the Russian novelist Turgenieff weighed 2,012), the brains of many eminent men are not distinguished for their great size. That of the French statesman Gambetta weighed only 1,160 grams. It must be borne in mind also that there are many individuals among the lower races and among women having brain weight much in excess of that of that of the average male white.

Of all the possible ways of treating the brain for the purpose of testing its intelligence, that of weighing is the least satisfactory, and has been most indefatigably practiced. A better method, that of counting the nerve cells, has been lately introduced, but to treat a single brain in this way is a work of years, and no series of results exists. In the meantime Miss Thompson, in co-operation with Professor Angell, has completed a study of the mental traits of men and women on what is perhaps the best available principle— that of a series of laboratory tests which eliminate or take into consideration differences due to the characteristic habits of the two sexes. Her findings are probably the most important contribution in this field, and her general conclusion on differences of sex will, I think, hold also for differences of race:

> The point to be emphasized as the outcome of this study is that, according to our present light, the psychological differences of sex seem to be largely due, not to difference of average capacity, nor to difference in type of mental activity, but to differences in the social influences brought to bear on the developing individual from early infancy to adult years. The question of the future development of the intellectual life of women is one of social necessities and ideals rather than of the inborn psychological characteristics of sex.[258]

There is certainly great difference in the mental ability of individuals, and there are probably less marked differences in the average ability of different races; but difference in natural ability is, in the main, a characteristic of the individual, not of race or of sex. It is probable that brain efficiency (speaking from the biological standpoint) has been, on the average, approximately the same in all races and in both sexes since nature first made up a good working-model, and that differences in intellectual expression are mainly social rather than biological, dependent on the fact that different stages of culture present different experiences to the mind, and adventitious circumstances direct the attention to different fields of interest.

II

In approaching the question of the parity or disparity of the mental ability of the white and the lower races, we bring to it a fixed and instinctive prejudice. No race views another race with that generosity with which it views itself. It may even be said that the existence of a social group depends on its taking an exaggerated view of its own importance; and in a state of nature, at least, the same is true of the individual. If self-preservation is the first law of nature, there must be on the mental side an acute consciousness of self, and a habit of regarding the self as of more importance than the world at large. The value of this standpoint lies in the fact that, while a wholesome fear of the enemy is important, a wholesome contempt is even more so. Praising one's self and dispraising an antagonist creates a confidence and a mental superiority in the way of confidence. The vituperative recriminations of modern prize-fighters, the boastings of the Homeric heroes, and the *bôgan* of the old Germans, like the back-talk of the small boy, were calculated to screw the courage up; and the Indians of America usually gave a dance before going on the war-path, in which by pantomime and boasting they magnified themselves and their past, and so stimulated their self-esteem that they felt invincible. In race-prejudice we see the same tendency to exalt the self and the group at the expense of outsiders. The alien group is belittled by attaching contempt to its peculiarities and habits—its color, speech, dress, and all the signs of its personality. This is not a laudable attitude, but it has been valuable to the group, because a bitter and contemptuous feeling is an aid to good fighting.

No race or nation has yet freed itself from this tendency to exalt and idealize itself. It is very difficult for a member of western civilization to understand that the orientals regard us with a contempt in comparison with which our contempt for them is feeble. Our bloodiness, our newness, our lack of reverence, our land-greed, our break-neck speed and lack of appreciation of leisure make Vandals of us. On the other hand, we are very stupid about recognizing the intelligence of orientals. We have been accustomed to think that there is a great gulf between ourselves and other races; and this persists in an undefinable way after scores of Japanese have taken high rank in our schools, and after Hindus have repeatedly been among the wranglers in mathematics at Cambridge. It is only when one of the far eastern nations has come bodily to the front that we begin to ask ourselves whether there is not an error in our reckoning.

The instinct to belittle outsiders is perhaps at the bottom of our delusion that the white race has one order of mind and the black and yellow races have another. But, while a prejudice—a matter of instinct and emotion—may well be at the beginning of an error of this kind, it could not sustain itself in the face of our logical habits unless reinforced by an error of the judgment. And this error is found in the fact that in a naïve way we assume that our steps in progress from time to time are due to our mental superiority as a race over other races, and to the mental superiority of one generation of ourselves over the preceding.

In this we are confusing advance in culture with brain improvement. If we should assume a certain grade of intelligence, fixed and invariable in all individuals, races, and times—an unwarranted assumption, of course— progress would still be possible, provided we assumed a characteristically human grade of intelligence to begin with. With associative memory, abstraction, and speech men are able to compare the present with the past, to deliberate and discuss, to invent, to abandon old processes for new, to focus attention on special problems, to encourage specialization, and to transmit to the younger generation a more intelligent standpoint and a more advanced starting-point. Culture is the accumulation of the results of activity, and culture could go on improving for a certain time even if there were a retrogression in intelligence. If all the chemists in class A should stop work tomorrow, the chemists in class B would still make discoveries. These would influence manufacture, and progress would result. If a worker in any specialty acquaints himself with the results of his predecessors and contemporaries and *works*, he will add some results to the sum of knowledge in his line. And if a race preserves by record or tradition the memory of what past generations have done, and adds a little, progress is secured whether the brain improves or stands still. In the same way, the fact that one race has advanced farther in culture than another does not necessarily imply a different order of brain, but may be due to the fact that in the one case social arrangements have not taken the shape affording the most favorable conditions for the operation of the mind.

If, then, we make due allowance for our instinctive tendency as a white group to disparage outsiders, and, on the other hand, for our tendency to confuse progress in culture and general intelligence with biological modification of the brain, we shall have to reduce very much our usual estimate of the difference in mental capacity between ourselves and the lower races, if we do not eliminate it altogether; and we shall perhaps have to abandon altogether the view that there has been an increase in the mental capacity of the white race since prehistoric times.

The first question arising in this connection is whether any of the characteristic faculties of the human mind—perception, memory, inhibition, abstraction—are absent or noticeably weak in the lower races. If this is found to be true, we have reason to attribute the superiority of the white race to biological causes; otherwise we shall have to seek an explanation of white superiority in causes lying outside the brain.

In examining this question we need not dwell on the acuteness of the sense-perceptions, because these are not distinctively human. As a matter of fact, they are usually better developed in animals and in the lower races than in the civilized, because the lower mental life is more perceptive than ratiocinative. The memory of the lower races is also apparently quite as good as that of the higher. The memory of the Australian native or the Eskimo is quite as good as that of our "oldest inhabitant;" and probably no one would claim that the modern scientist has a better memory than the bard of the Homeric period.

There is, however, a prevalent view, for the popularization of which Herbert Spencer is largely responsible, that primitive man has feeble powers of inhibition. Like the equally erroneous view that early man is a free and unfettered creature, it arises from our habit of assuming that, because his inhibitions and unfreedom do not correspond with our own restraints, they do not exist. Sir John Lubbock pointed out long ago that the savage is hedged about by conventions so minute and so mandatory that he is actually the least free person in the world. But, in spite of this, Spencer and others have insisted that he is incapable of self-restraint, is carried away like a child by the impulse of the moment, and is incapable of rejecting an immediate gratification for a greater future one. Cases like the one mentioned by Darwin of the Fuegian who struck and killed his little son when the latter dropped a basket of fish into the water are cited without regard to the fact that cases of sudden domestic violence and quick repentance are common in any city today; and the failure of the Australian blacks to throw back the small fry when seining is referred to without pausing to consider that our practice of exterminating game and denuding our forests shows an amazing lack of individual self-restraint.

The truth is that the restraints exercised in a group depend largely on the traditions, views, and teachings of the group, and, if we have this in mind, the savage cannot be called deficient on the side of inhibition. It is doubtful if modern society affords anything more striking in the way of inhibition than is found in connection with taboo, fetish, totemism, and ceremonial among the lower races. In the great majority of the American Indian and Australian tribes a man is strictly forbidden to kill or eat the animals whose name his clan bears as a totem. The central Australian may not, in addition, eat the flesh of any animal killed or even touched by persons standing in certain relations of kinship to him. At certain times also he is forbidden to eat the flesh of a number of animals and at all times he must share all food secured with the tribal elders and some others.

A native of Queensland will put his mark on an unripe zamia fruit, and may be sure that it will be untouched and that when it is ripe he has only to go and get it. The Eskimos, though starving, will not molest the sacred seal basking before their huts. Similarly in social intercourse the inhibitions are numerous. To some of his sisters, blood and tribal, the Australian may not speak at all; to others only at certain distances, according to the degree of kinship. The west African fetish acts as a police, and property protected by it is safer than under civilized laws. Food and palm wine are placed beside the path with a piece of fetish suspended near by, and no one will touch them without leaving the proper payment. The garden of a native may be a mile from the house, unfenced, and sometimes unvisited for weeks by the owner; but it is immune from depredations if protected by fetish. Our proverb says, "A hungry belly has no ears," and it must be admitted that the inhibition of food impulses implies no small power of restraint.

Altogether too much has been made of inhibition, anyway, as a sign of mentality, for it is not even characteristic of the human species. The well-trained dog inhibits in the presence of the most enticing stimulations of the kitchen. And it is also true that one race, at least—the American Indian—makes inhibition of the most conspicuous feature in its system of education. From the time the ice is broken to give him a cold plunge and begin the toughening process on the day of his birth, until he dies with out a groan under torture the Indian is schooled in the restraint of his impulses. He does not, indeed, practice our identical restraints, because his traditions and the run of his attention are different; but he has a capacity for controlling impulse equal to our own.

Another serious charge against the intelligence of the lower races is lack of the power of abstraction. They certainly do not deal largely in abstraction, and their languages are poor in abstract terms. But there is a great difference between the habit of thinking in abstract terms and the ability to do so.

The degree to which abstraction is employed in the activities of a group depends on the complexity of the activities and on the complexity of consciousness in the group. When science, philosophy, and logic, and systems of reckoning time, space, and number are taught in the schools; when the attention is not so much engaged in perceptual as in deliberate acts; and when thought is a profession, then abstract modes of thought are forced on the mind. This does not argue absence of the power of abstraction in the lower races, or even a low grade of ability, but lack of practice. To one skilled in any line an unpracticed person seems very stupid; and this is apparently the reason why travelers report that the black and yellow races have feeble powers of abstraction. It is generally admitted, however, that the use of speech involves the power of abstraction, so that all races have the power in some degree. When we come further to examine the degree in which they possess it, we find that they compare favorably with ourselves in any test which involves a fair comparison.

The proverb is a form of abstraction practiced by all races, and is perhaps the best test of the natural bent of the mind in this direction, because, like ballad poetry, and slang, proverbial sayings do not originate with the educated class, but are of popular origin. At the same time, proverbs compare favorably with the *mots* of literature, and many proverbs have, in fact, drifted into literature and become connected with the names of great writers. Indeed, the saying that there is nothing new under the sun applies with such force and fidelity to literature that, if we should strip Hesiod and Homer and Chaucer of such phrases as "The half is greater than the whole," "It is a wise son that knows his own father" (which Shakespeare quotes the other end about), and "To make a virtue of necessity," and if we should further eliminate from literature the motives and sentiments also in ballad poetry and in popular thought, little would remain but form.

If we assume, then, that the popular mind—let us say the peasant mind—in the white race is as capable of abstraction as the mind of the higher classes, but not so specialized in this direction—and no one can doubt this in view of the academic record of country-bred boys—the following comparison of our proverbs with those of the Africans of the Guinea coast (the latter reported by the late Sir A.B. Ellis[259]) is significant:

African. Stone in the water-hole does not feel the cold.
English. Habit is second nature.

A. One tree does not make a forest.
E. One swallow does not make a summer.

A. "I nearly killed the bird." No one can eat nearly in a stew.
E. First catch your hare.

A. Full-belly child says to hungry-belly child, "Keep good cheer."
E. We can all endure the misfortunes of others.

A. Distant firewood is good firewood.
E. Distance lends enchantment to the view.

A. Ashes fly back in the face of him who throws them.
E. Curses come home to roost.

A. If the boy says he wants to tie the water with a string, ask him whether he
    means the water in the pot or the water in the lagoon.
E. Answer a fool according to his folly.

A. Cowries are men.
E. Money makes the man.

A. Cocoanut is not good for bird to eat.
E. Sour grapes.

A. He runs away from the sword and hides himself in the scabbard.
E. Out of the frying-pan into the fire.

A. A fool of Ika and an idiot of Iluka meet together to make friends.
E. Birds of a feather flock together.

A. The ground-pig [bandicoot] said: "I do not feel so angry with the man
    who killed me as with the man who dashed me on the ground
    afterward."
E. Adding insult to injury.

A. Quick loving a woman means quick not loving a woman.
E. Married in haste we repent at leisure.

A. Three elders cannot all fail to pronounce the word *ekulu* [an antelope]:
    one may say *ekúlu*, another *ekulú*, but the third will say *ekulu*.
E. In a multitude of counselors there is safety.

A. If the stomach is not strong, do not eat cockroaches.
E. Milk for babes.

A. No one should draw water from the spring in order to supply the river.
E. Robbing Peter to pay Paul.

A. The elephant makes a dust and the buffalo makes a dust, but the dust of the buffalo is lost in the dust of the elephant.
E. Duo cum faciunt idem non est idem.

A. Ear, hear the other before you decide.
E. Audi alteram partem.

On the side of number we have another test of the power of abstraction; and while the lower races show lack of practice in this, they show no lack of power. It is true that tribes have been found with no names for numbers beyond two, three, or five; but these are isolated groups, like the Veddahs and Bushmen, who have no trade or commerce, and lead a miserable existence, with little or nothing to count. The directions of attention and the simplicity or complexity of mental processes depend on the character of the external situation which the mind has to manipulate. If the activities are simple, the mind is simple, and if the activities were nil, the mind would be nil. The mind is nothing but a means of manipulating the outside world. Number, time, and space conceptions and systems become more complex and accurate, not as the human mind grows in capacity, but as activities become more varied and call for more extended and accurate systems of notation and measurement. Trade and commerce, machinery and manufacture, and all the processes of civilization involve specialization in the apprehension of series as such. Under these conditions the number technique becomes elaborate and requires time and instruction for its mastery. The advance which mathematics has made within a brief historical time is strikingly illustrated by the words with which the celebrated mathematician, Sir Henry Savile, who died in 1662, closed his career as a professor at Oxford:

> By the grace of God, gentlemen hearers, I have performed my promise. I have redeemed my pledge. I have explained, according to my ability, the definitions, postulates, axioms, and the first eight

propositions of the *Elements* of Euclid. Here, sinking under the weight of years, I lay down my art and my instruments.[260]

From the standpoint of modern mathematics, Sir Henry Savile and the Bushman are both woefully backward; and in both cases the backwardness is not a matter of mental incapacity, but of the state of the science.

In respect, then, to brain structure and the more important mental faculties we find that no race is radically unlike the others. Still, it might happen that the mental activities and products of two groups were so different as to place them in different classes. But precisely the contrary is true. There is in force a principle called the law of parallelism in development, according to which any group takes much the same steps in development as any other. The group may be belated, indeed, and not reach certain stages, but the ground patterns of life are the same in the lower races and in the higher. Mechanical inventions, textile industries, rude painting, poetry, sculpture, and song, marriage and family life, organization under leaders, belief in spirits, a mythology, and some form of church and state exist universally. At one time students of mankind, when they found a myth in Hawaii corresponding to the Greek story of Orpheus and Eurydice, or an Aztec poem of tender longing in absence, or a story of the deluge, were wont to conjecture how these could have been carried over from Greek or Elizabethan or Hebraic sources, or whether they did not afford evidence of a time when all branches of the human race dwelt together with a common fund of sentiment and tradition. But this standpoint has been abandoned, and it is recognized that the human mind and the outside world are essentially alike the world over; that the mind everywhere acts on the same principles; and that, ignoring the local, incidental, and eccentric, we find similar laws of growth among all peoples.

The number of things which can stimulate the human mind is somewhat definite and limited. Among them, for example, is death. This happens everywhere, and the death of a dear one may cause the living to imagine ways of being reunited. The story of Orpheus and Eurydice may thus arise spontaneously and perpetually, wherever death and affection exist. Or, there may be a separation from home and friends, and the mind runs back in distress and longing over the happy past, and the state of consciousness aroused is as definite a fact among savages as among the civilized. A beautiful passage in Homer represents Helen looking out on the Greeks from the wall of Troy and saying:

> And now behold I all the other glancing-eyed Achaians, whom well I could discern and tell their names; but two captains of the host can I not see, even Kastor tamer of horses and Polydukes the skilful boxer, mine own brethren whom the same mother bare. Either they came not in the company from lovely Lakedaimon; or they came hither indeed in their seafaring ships, but now will not enter into the battle of the warriors, for fear of the many scornings and revilings that are mine.[261]

When this passage is thus stripped of its technical excellence by a prose translation, we may compare it with the following New Zealand lament composed by a young woman who was captured on the island of Tuhua and carried to a mountain from which she could see her home:

> My regret is not to be expressed. Tears, like a spring, gush from my eyes. I wonder whatever is Tu Kainku [her lover] doing, he who deserted me. Now I climb upon the ridge of Mount Parahaki, whence is clear the view of the island of Tuhua. I see with regret the lofty Tanmo where dwells [the chief] Tangiteruru. If I were there, the shark's tooth would hang from my ear. How fine, how beautiful should I look!... But enough of this; I must return to my rags and to my nothing at all.[262]

The situation of the two women in this case is not identical, and it would be possible to claim that the Greek and Maori passages differ in tone and coloring; but it remains true that a captive woman of any race will feel much the same as a captive woman of any other race when her thoughts turn toward home, and that the poetry growing out of such a situation will be everywhere of the same general pattern.

Similarly, to take an illustration from morals, we find that widely different in complexion and detail as are the moral codes of lower and higher groups, say the Hebrews and the African Kafirs, yet the general patterns of morality are strikingly coincident. It is reported of the Kafirs that "they possess laws which meet every crime which may be committed." Theft is punished by restitution and fine; injuring cattle, by death or fine; false witness, by a heavy fine; adultery, by fine or death; rape, by fine or death; poisoning or witchcraft, by death and confiscation of property; murder, by death or fine; treason or desertion from the tribe, by death or confiscation.[263] The Kafirs and Hebrews are not at the same level of culture, and we miss the more abstract and monotheistic admonitions of the higher religion—"thou shalt not covet; thou shalt worship no other gods before me"—but the intelligence shown by the social mind in adjusting the individual to society may fairly be called the same grade of intelligence in the two cases.

When the environmental life of two groups is more alike and the general cultural conditions more correspondent, the parallelism of thought and practice becomes more striking. The recently discovered Assyrian Code of Hammurabi (about 2500 B.C.) contains striking correspondences with the Mosaic code; and while Semitic scholars probably have good and sufficient reasons for holding that the Mosaic Code was strongly influenced by the Assyrian, we may yet be very confident that the two codes would have been of the same general character if no influence whatever had passed from one to the other.

The institutions and practices of a people are a product of the mind; and if the early and spontaneous products of mind are everywhere of the same general pattern as the later manifestations, only less developed, refined, and specialized, it may well be that failure to progress equally is not due to essential unlikeness of mind, but to conditions lying outside the mind.

Another test of mental ability which deserves special notice is mechanical ingenuity. Our white pre-eminence owes much to this faculty, and the lower races are reckoned defective in it. But the lower races do invent, and it is doubtful whether one invention is ever much more difficult than another. On the psychological side, an invention means that the mind sees a roundabout way of reaching an end when it cannot be reached directly. It brings into play the associative memory, and involves the recognition of analogies. There is a certain likeness between the flying back of a bough in one's face and the rebound of a bow, between a serpent's tooth and a poisoned arrow, between floating timber and a raft or boat; and water, steam, and electricity are like a horse in one respect—they will all make wheels go around, and do work.

Now, the savage had this faculty of seeing analogies and doing things in indirect ways. With the club, knife, and sword he struck more effectively than with the fist; with hooks, traps, nets, and pitfalls he understood how to seize game more surely than with the hands; in the bow and arrow, spear, blow-gun, and spring-trap he devised motion swifter than that of his own body; he protected himself with armor imitated from the hides and scales of animals, and turned their venom back on themselves. That the savage should have originated the inventive process and carried it on systematically is, indeed, more wonderful than that his civilized successors should continue the process; for every beginning is difficult.

When occupations become specialized and one set of men has continually to do with one and only one set of machinery and forces, the constant play of attention over the limited field naturally results in improvements and the introduction of new principles. Modern inventions are magnificent and seem quite to overshadow the simpler devices of primitive times; but when we consider the precedents, copies, resources, and accumulated knowledge with which the modern investigator works, and, on the other hand, the resourcelessness of primitive man in materials, ideas, and in the inventive habit itself, I confess that the bow and arrow seems to me the most wonderful invention in the world.

Viewing the question from a different angle, we find another argument for the homogeneous character of the human mind in the fact that the patterns of interest of the civilized show no variation from those of the savage. Not only the appetites and vanities remain essentially the same, but, on the side of intellectual interest, the type of mental reaction fixed in the savage by the food-quest has come down unaltered to the man of science as well as to the man of the street. In circumventing enemies and capturing game, both the attention and the organic processes worked together in primitive man under great stress and strain. Whenever, indeed, a strain is thrown on the attention, the heart and organs of respiration are put under pressure also in their effort to assist the attention in manipulating the problem; and these organic fluctuations are felt as pleasure and pain. The strains thrown on the attention of primitive man were connected with his struggle for life; and not only in the actual encounter with men and animals did emotion run high, but the memory and anticipation of conflict reinstated the emotional conditions in those periods when he was meditating future conflicts and preparing his bows and arrows, traps and poisons. The problem of invention, the reflective and scientific side of his life, was suffused with interest, because the manufacture of the weapon was, psychologically speaking, a part of the fight.

This type of interest, originating in the hunt, remains dominant in the mind down to the present time. Once constructed to take an interest in the hunting problem, it takes an interest in any problem whatever. Not only do hunting and fighting and all competitive games—which are of precisely the same psychological pattern as the hunt and fight—remain of perennial interest, but all the useful occupations are interesting in just the degree that this pattern is preserved. The man of science works at problems and uses his ingenuity in making an engine in the laboratory in the same way that primitive man used his mind in making a trap. So long as the problem is present, the interest is sustained; and the interest ceases when the problematical is removed. Consequently, all modern occupations of the hunting pattern—scientific investigation, law, medicine, the organization of business, trade speculation, and the arts and crafts—are interesting as a game; while those occupations into which the division of labor enters to the degree that the workman is not attempting to control a problem, and in which the same acts are repeated an indefinite number of times, lose interest and become extremely irksome.

This means that the brain acts pleasurably on the principle it was made up to act on in the most primitive times, and the rest is a burden. There is no brain change, but the social changes have been momentous; and the brain of each generation is brought into contact with new traditions, inhibitions, copies, obligations, problems, so that the run of attention and content of consciousness are different. Social suggestion works marvels in the manipulation of the mind; but the change is not in the brain as an organ; it is rather in the character of the stimulations thrust on it by society.

The child begins as a savage, and after we have brought to bear all the influence of home, school, and church to socialize him, we speak as though his nature had changed organically, and institute a parallelism between the child and the race, assuming that the child's brain passes in a recapitulatory way through phases of development corresponding to epochs in the history of the race. I have no doubt myself that this theory of recapitulation is largely a misapprehension. A stream of social influence is turned loose on the child; and if the attention to him is incessant and wise, and the copies he has are good and stimulating, he is molded nearer to the heart's desire. Sometimes he escapes, and becomes a criminal, tramp, sport, or artist; and even if made into an impeccable and model citizen, he periodically breaks away from the network of social habit and goes a-fishing.

The fundamental explanation of the difference in the mental life of two groups is not that the capacity of the brain to do work is different, but that the attention is not in the two cases stimulated and engaged along the same lines. Wherever society furnishes copies and stimulations of a certain kind, a body of knowledge and a technique, practically all its members are able to work on the plan and scale in vogue there, and members of an alien race who become acquainted in a real sense with the system can work under it. But when society does not furnish the stimulations, or when it has preconceptions which tend to inhibit the run of attention in given lines, then the individual shows no intelligence in these lines. This may be illustrated in the fields of scientific and artistic interest. Among the Hebrews a religious inhibition—"thou shalt not make unto thee any graven image"—was sufficient to prevent anything like the sculpture of the Greeks; and the doctrine of the resurrection of the body in the early Christian church, and the teaching that man was made in the image of God, formed an almost insuperable obstacle to the study of human anatomy.

The Mohammedan attitude toward scientific interest is represented by the following extracts from a letter from an oriental official to a western inquirer, printed by Sir Austen Henry Layard:

My Illustrious Friend and Joy of my Liver:

The thing which you ask of me is both difficult and useless. Although I have passed all my days in this place, I have neither counted the houses nor inquired into the number of the inhabitants; and as to what one person loads on his mules and the other stows away in the bottom of his ship, that is no business of mine. But above all, as to the previous history of this city, God only knows the amount of dirt and confusion that the infidels may have eaten before the coming of the sword of Islam. It were unprofitable for us to inquire into it.... Listen, O my son! There is no wisdom equal to the belief in God! He created the world, and shall we liken ourselves unto him in seeking to penetrate into the mysteries of his creation? Shall we say, Behold this star spinneth round that star, and this other star with a tail goeth and cometh in so many years? Let it go! He from whose hand it came will guide and direct it.... Thou art learned in the things I care not for, and as for that which thou hast seen, I spit upon it. Will much knowledge create thee a double belly, or wilt thou seek paradise with thine eyes?...

The meek in spirit,
IMAUM ALI ZADI.[264]

The works of Sir Henry Maine, who gained by his long residence in India a profound insight into the oriental character, frequently point out that the eastern pride in conservatisms is quite as real as the western pride in progress:

> Vast populations, some of them with a civilization considerable but peculiar, detest that which in the language of the West would be called reform. The entire Mohammedan world detests it. The multitudes of colored men who swarm in the great continent of Africa detest it, and it is detested by that large part of mankind which we are accustomed to leave on one side as barbarous or savage. The millions upon millions of men who fill the Chinese Empire loathe it and (what is more) despise it.... There are few things more remarkable, and in their way more instructive, than the stubborn incredulity and disdain which a man belonging to the cultivated part of Chinese society opposes to the vaunts of western civilization which he frequently hears.... There is in India a minority, educated at the feet of English politicians and in books saturated with English political ideas, which has learned to repeat their language; but it is doubtful whether even these, if they had

a voice in the matter, would allow a finger to be laid on the very subjects with which European legislation is beginning to concern itself —social and religious usage. There is not, however, the shadow of a doubt that the enormous mass of the Indian population hates and dreads change.[265]

To the fact that the enthusiasm for change is comparatively rare must be added the fact that it is extremely modern. It is known but to a small part of mankind, and to that part but for a short period during a history of incalculable length.[266]

The oriental attitude does not argue a lack of brain power, but a prepossession hostile to scientific inquiry. The society represented does not interest its members in what, from the western standpoint, is knowledge.

The Chinese afford a fine example of a people of great natural ability letting their intelligence run to waste from lack of a scientific standpoint. As indicated above, they are not defective in brain weight, and their application to study is long continued and very severe; but their attention is directed to matters which cannot possibly make them wise from the occidental standpoint. They learn no mathematics and no science, but spend years in copying the poetry of the T'ang Dynasty, in order to learn the Chinese characters, and in the end cannot write the language correctly, because many modern characters are not represented in this ancient poetry. Their attention to Chinese history is great, as befits their reverence for the past; but they do not organize their knowledge, they have no adequate textbooks or apparatus for study, and they make no clear distinction between fact and fiction. In general, they learn only rules and no principles, and rely on memory without the aid of reason, with the result that the man who stops studying often forgets everything, and the professional student is amazingly ignorant in the line of his own work:

Multitudes of Chinese scholars know next to nothing about matters directly in the line of their studies, and in regard to which we should consider ignorance positively disgraceful. A venerable teacher remarked to the writer with a charming naïveté that he had never understood the allusions in the Trimetrical Classic (which stands at the very threshold of Chinese study) until at the age of sixty he had an opportunity to read a Universal History prepared by a missionary, in which for the first time Chinese history was made accessible to him.[267]

Add to this that the whole of their higher learning, corresponding to our university system, consists in writing essays and always more essays on the Chinese classics, and "it is impossible," as Mr. Smith points out, "not to marvel at the measure of success which has attended the use of such materials in China."[268] But when this people is in possession of the technique of the western world—a logic, general ideas, and experimentation—we cannot reasonably doubt that they will be able to work the western system as their cousins, the Japanese, are doing, and perhaps they, too, may better the instruction.

White effectiveness is probably due to a superior technique acting in connection with a superior body of knowledge and sentiment. Of two groups having equal mental endowment, one may outstrip the other by the mere dominance of incident. It is a notorious fact that the course of human history has been largely without prevision or direction. Things have drifted and forces have arisen. Under these conditions an unusual incident—the emergence of a great mind or a forcible personality, or the operation of influences as subtle as those which determine fashions in dress—may establish social habits and duties which will give a distinct character to the modes of attention and mental life of the group. The most significant fact for Aryan development is the emergence among the Greeks of a number of eminent men who developed logic, the experimental method, and philosophic interest, and fixed in their group the habit of looking behind the incident for the general law. Mediaeval attention was diverted from these lines by a religious movement, and the race lost for a time the key to progress and got clean away from the Greek copies; but it found them again and took a fresh start with the revival of Greek learning. It is quite possible to make a fetish of classical learning; but Sir Henry Maine's remark, that nothing moves in the modern world that is not Greek in its origin, is quite just.

The real variable is the individual, not the race. In the beginning—perhaps as the result of a mutation or series of mutations—a type of brain developed which has remained relatively fixed in all times and among all races. This brain will never have any faculty in addition to what it now possesses, because as a type of structure it is as fixed as the species itself, and is indeed a mark of species. It is not apparent either that we are greatly in need of another faculty, or that we could make use of it even if by a chance mutation it should emerge, since with the power of abstraction we are able to do any class of work we know anything about. Moreover, the brain is less likely to make a leap now than in earlier time, both because the conditions of nature are more fixed or more nearly controlled by man, and hence the urgency of adjustment to sharp variations in external conditions is removed, and because the struggle for existence has been mitigated so that the unfit survive along with the fit. Indeed, the rapid increase in idiocy and insanity shown by statistics indicates that the brain is deteriorating slightly, *on the average*, as compared with earlier times.[269]

Nature is not producing a better average brain than in the time of Aristotle and the Greeks. If we have more than the wisdom of our ancestors, our advantage lies in our specialization, our superior body of knowledge, and our superior technique for its transmission. At the same time, the individual brain is unstable, fluctuating in normal persons between 1,100 and 1,500 grams in weight, while the extremes of variation are represented, on the one side, by the imbecile with 300 grams, and the man of genius with 2,000 on the other. It is therefore perfectly true that by artificial selection—Mr. Galton's "eugenism"—a larger average brain could be created, and also a higher average of natural intelligence, whether this be absolutely dependent on brain weight or not. But it is hardly to be expected that a stable brain above the capacity of those of the first rank now and in the past will result, since the mutations of nature are more radical than the breeding process of man, and she probably ran the whole gamut. "Great men lived before Agamemnon," and individual variations will continue to occur, but not on a different pattern; and what has been true in the past will happen again in the future, that the group which by hook or by crook comes into possession of the best technique and the best copies will make the best show of intelligence and march at the head of civilization.

III

The foregoing examination of the relation of the mental faculty of the lower races to the higher places us in a position to examine to better advantage the other question of the relation of the intelligence of woman to that of man.

The differences in mental expression between the lower and the higher races can be expressed for the most part in terms of attention and practice. The differences in run of attention and practice are in this case due to the development of different habits by groups occupying different habitats, and consequently having no copies in common. Woman, on the other hand, exists in the white man's world of practical and scientific activity, but is excluded from full participation in it. Certain organic conditions and historical incidents have, in fact, inclosed her in habits which she neither can nor will fracture, and have also set up in the mind of man an attitude toward her which renders her almost as alien to man's interests and practices as if she were spatially separated from them.

One of the most important facts which stand out in a comparison of the physical traits of men and women is that man is a more specialized instrument for motion, quicker on his feet, with a longer reach, and fitted for bursts of energy; while woman has a greater fund of stored energy and is consequently more fitted for endurance. The development of intelligence and motion have gone along side by side in all animal forms. Through motion chances and experiences are multiplied, the whole equilibrium characterizing the stationary form is upset, and the organs of sense and the intelligence are developed to take note of and manipulate the outside world. Amid the recurrent dangers incident to a world peopled with moving and predacious forms, two attitudes may be assumed—that of fighting, and that of fleeing or hiding. As between the two, concealment and evasion became more characteristic of the female, especially among mammals, where the young are particularly helpless and need protection for a long period. She remained, therefore, more stationary, and at the same time acquired more cunning, than the male.

In mankind especially, the fact that woman had to rely on cunning and the protection of man rather than on swift motion, while man had a freer range of motion and adopted a fighting technique, was the starting-point of a differentiation in the habits and interests, which had a profound effect on the consciousness of each. Man's most immediate, most fascinating, and most remunerative occupation was the pursuit of animal life. The pursuit of this stimulated him to the invention of devices for killing and capture; and this aptitude for invention was later extended to the invention of tools and of mechanical devices in general, and finally developed into a settled habit of scientific interest. The scientific imagination which characterizes man in contrast with women is not a distinctive male trait, but represents a constructive habit of attention associated with freer movement and the pursuit of evasive animal forms. The problem of control was more difficult, and the means of securing it became more indirect, mediated, reflective, and inventive; that is, more intelligent.

Woman's activities, on the other hand, were largely limited to plant life, to her children, and to manufacture, and the stimulation to mental life and invention in connection with these was not so powerful as in the case of man. Her inventions were largely processes of manufacture connected with her handling of the by-products of the chase. So simple a matter, therefore, as relatively unrestricted motion on the part of man and relatively restricted motion on the part of woman determined the occupations of each, and these occupations in turn created the characteristic mental life of each. In man this was constructive, answering to his varied experience and the need of controlling a moving environment; and in woman it was conservative, answering to her more stationary and monotonous condition.

In early times man's superior physical force, the wider range of his experience, his mechanical inventions in connection with hunting and fighting, and his combination under leadership with his comrades to carry out their common enterprises, resulted in a contempt for the weakness of women and an almost complete separation in interest between himself and the women of the group. The men frequently formed clubs, and lived apart from the women; and even where this did not happen, the men and women had no mental life in common. To this contempt for women also was added a superstitious fear of them, growing out of the primitive belief that weakness or any other bad quality is infectious, and may be transferred by physical contact or association.[270]

From Mr. Crawley's excellent paper on "Sexual Taboo" I transcribe the following illustrations of this attitude:

In New Caledonia you rarely see men and women talking or sitting together. The women seem perfectly content with the company of their own sex. The men who loiter about with spears in most lazy fashion are seldom seen in the society of the opposite sex.... The Ojebwey, Peter Jones, thus writes of his own people: "I have scarcely ever seen anything like social intercourse between husband and wife, and it is remarkable that the women say little in the presence of the men." The Zulus regard their women with a haughty contempt. If a man were going to the bush to cut firewood with his wives, he and they would take different paths, and neither go nor return in company. If he were going to visit a neighbor and wished his wife to go also, she would follow at a distance. In Senegambia the women live by themselves, rarely with their husbands, and their sex is virtually a clique. In Egypt a man never converses with his wife, and in the tomb they are separated by a wall, though males and females are not usually buried in the same vault.[271]

Amongst the Dacotas custom and superstition ordain that the wife must carefully keep away from all that belongs to her husband's sphere of action. The Bechuanas never allow their women to touch their cattle; accordingly the men have to plow themselves.... In Guiana no woman may go near the hut where *ourali* is made. In the Marquesas Islands the use of canoes is prohibited to the female sex by *tabu*: the breaking of the rule is punished with death. Conversely, amongst the same people *tapa*-making belongs exclusively to the women: when they are making it for their own headdresses it is *tabu* for the men to touch it. In Nicaragua all the marketing was done by the women. A man might not enter the market nor even see the proceedings at the risk of a beating.... In Samoa where the manufacture of cloth is allotted solely to the women, it is a degradation for a man to engage in any detail of the process.... An Eskimo thinks it an indignity to row in an *umiak*, the large boat used by women. The different offices of husband and wife are also clearly distinguished; for example, when he has brought his booty to land it would be a stigma on his character if he so much as drew a seal ashore, and generally it is regarded as scandalous for a man to interfere with what is the work of women. In British Guiana cooking is the province of the women, as elsewhere; on one occasion when the men were compelled perforce to bake some bread they were only persuaded to do so with the utmost difficulty, and were ever after pointed at as old women.[272]

Amongst the Barea, man and wife seldom share the same bed; the reason they give is that the breath of the wife weakens the husband.... The Khyoungthas have a legend of a man who reduced a king and his men to a condition of feebleness by persuading them to dress up as women and perform female duties. When they had thus been rendered effeminate they were attacked and defeated without a blow.... Contempt for female timidity has caused a curious custom amongst the Gallas: they amputate the mammae of the boys soon after birth, believing that no warrior can possibly be brave who possesses them, and that they should belong to women only.... Amongst the Lhoosais when a man is unable to do his work, whether through laziness, cowardice or bodily incapacity, he is dressed in women's clothes and has to associate and work with the women. Amongst the Pomo Indians of California, when a man becomes too infirm for a warrior he is made a menial and assists the squaws.... When the Delawares were denationized by the Iroquois and prohibited from going to war they were according to the Indian notion "made women," and were henceforth to confine themselves to the pursuits appropriate to women.[273]

Women were still further degraded by the development of property and its control by man, together with the habit of treating her as a piece of property, whose value was enhanced if its purity was assured and demonstrable. As a result of this situation, man's chief concern in women became an interest in securing the finest specimens for his own use, in guarding them with jealous care from contact with other men, and in making them, together with the ornaments they wore, signs of his wealth and social standing. The instances below are extreme ones, taken from lower social stages than our own, but they differ only in degree from the chaperonage of modern Europe:

I heard from a teacher about some strange custom connected with some of the young girls here [New Ireland], so I asked the chief to take me to the house where they were. The house was about twenty-five feet in length and stood in a reed and bamboo enclosure, across the entrance of which a bundle of dried grass was suspended to show that it was strictly *tabu*. Inside the house there were three conical structures about seven or eight feet in height, and about ten or twelve feet in circumference at the bottom, and for about four feet from the ground, at which point they tapered off to a point at the top. These cages were made of the broad leaves of the pandanus tree, sewn quite close together so that no light, and little or no air could enter. On one side of each is an opening which is closed by a double door of plaited cocoanut tree and pandanus tree leaves. About three feet from the ground there is a stage of bamboos which forms the floor. In each of these cages, we were told there was a young woman confined, each of whom had to remain for at least four or five years without ever being allowed to go outside the house. I could scarcely credit the story when I heard it; the whole thing seemed too horrible to be true. I spoke to the chief and told him that I wished to see the inside of the cages, and also to see the girls that I might make them a present of a few beads.... [A girl having been allowed to come out] I then went to inspect the inside of the cage out of which she had come, but could scarcely put my head inside of it, the atmosphere was so hot and stifling. It was clean and contained nothing but a few short lengths of bamboo for holding water. There was only room for the girl to sit or lie down in a crouched position on the bamboo platform, and when the doors are shut it must be nearly or quite dark inside. They are never allowed to come out except once a day to bathe in a dish or wooden bowl placed close to the cage. They say that they perspire profusely. They are placed in these stifling cages when quite young, and must remain there until they are young women, when they are taken out and have each a great marriage feast prepared for them. One of them was about fourteen or fifteen years old, and the chief told me that she had been there for five years, but would soon be taken out now. The other two were about eight and ten years old, and they have to stay there for several years longer. I asked if they never died, but they said "No."[274]

They [the Azande] are extremely jealous of their womenfolk, whom they do not permit to live in the same village with themselves. The women's village is generally in the bush, about 200 yards or so distant from that of the chief. Women are never seen in an Azande village, the pathway to their own being kept secret from all outsiders. This system while being something like that observed by the Arabs, has the important distinction that the women are not shut up. They are free to come and go and do what they like, except visit the men's village. In common with the entire native population of Central Africa, the custom among the Zande is that the men do no work that is not connected with the chase or the manufacture of implements. All agriculture is carried on by the women.[275]

From the time of engagement until marriage a young lady is required to maintain the strictest seclusion. Whenever friends call upon her parents she is expected to retire to the inner apartments, and in all her actions and words guard her conduct with careful solicitude. She must use a close sedan whenever she visits her relations, and in her intercourse with her brothers and the domestics in the household maintain great reserve. Instead of having any opportunity to form those friendships and acquaintances with her own sex which among ourselves become a source of much pleasure at the time and advantage in after life, the Chinese maiden is confined to the circle of her relations and her immediate neighbors. She has few of the pleasing remembrances and associations that are usually connected with school-day life, nor has she often the ability or opportunity to correspond by letter with girls of her own age. Seclusion at this time of life, and the custom of crippling the feet, combine to confine women in the house almost as much as the strictest laws against their appearing abroad; for in girlhood, as they know only a few persons except relatives, and can make very few acquaintances after marriage their circle of friends contracts rather than enlarges as life goes on. This privacy impels girls to learn as much of the world as they can, and among the rich their curiosity is gratified through maid-servants, match-makers, peddlers, visitors, and others.[276]

The world of white civilization is intellectually rich because it has amassed a rich fund of general ideas, and has organized these into specialized bodies of knowledge, and has also developed a special technique for the presentation of this knowledge and standpoint to the young members of society, and for localizing their attention in special fields of interest. When for any reason a class of society is excluded from this process, as women have been historically, it must necessarily remain ignorant. But, while no one would make any question that women confined as these in New Ireland and China, as shown above, must have an intelligence as restricted as their mode of life, we are apt to lose sight altogether of the fact that chivalry and chaperonage and modern convention are the persistence of the old race habit of contempt for women, and of their intellectual sequestration. Men and women still form two distinct classes and are not in free communication with each other. Not only are women unable and unwilling to be communicated with directly, unconventionally, and truly on many subjects, but men are unwilling to talk to them. I do not have in mind situations involving questions of propriety or delicacy alone, but a certain habit of restraint, originating doubtless in matters relating to sex, extends to all intercourse with women, with the result that they are not really admitted to the intellectual world of men; and there is not only a reluctance on the part of men to admit them, but a reluctance—or, rather, a real inability—on their part to enter. Modesty with reference to personal habits has become so ingrained and habitual, and to do anything freely is so foreign to woman, that even free thought is almost of the nature of an immodesty in her.

In connection also with the adventitious position of woman referred to in another paper,[277] the feminine interests and habits are set so strongly toward dress and personal display that they are not readily diverted. Women may and do protest against the triviality of their lives, but emotional interests are more immediate than intellectual ones, and human nature does not drift into intellectual pursuit voluntarily, but is forced into it in connection with the urgency of practical activities. The women who are obliged to work are of the poorer classes, and have not that leisure and opportunity preliminary to any specialized acquirement; while those who have leisure are supported in that position both by money and by precedent and habit, and have no immediate stimulation to lift them out of it. They sometimes entertain ideas of freedom and plan occupational interests, but they have usually become thoroughly habituated to their unfreedom, and continue to feed from the hand.

Custom lies upon them with a weight
Heavy as frost and deep almost as life.

The usual reasoning as to the ability of women also overlooks the fact that many women are larger and stronger than many men, and some of them possessed of tremendous energy, will, wit, endurance, and sagacity. This type appears in all classes of society, but more frequently in the lower classes and among peasants, both because the natural qualities are less glozed over there by aristocratic custom, and because these classes are bred truer to nature. Unfortunately, the attention of the women of these classes is limited to very immediate concerns; but, on the other hand, they present the true qualities of the female type, and few, I believe, will deny that the peasant woman described below would shine in intellectual walks if fate had called her there:

> Mother was a large, stout, full-blooded woman of great strength. She could not read or write, and yet she was well thought of. There are all sorts of educations, and though reading and writing are very well in their way, they would not have done mother any good. She had the sort of education that was needed in her work. Nobody knew more about raising vegetables, ducks, chickens and pigeons than she did. There were some among the neighbors who could read and write and so thought themselves above mother, but when they went to market they found their mistake. Her peas, beans, cauliflower, cabbages, pumpkins, melons, potatoes, beets, and onions sold for the highest price of any, and that ought to show whose education was the best, because it is the highest education that produces the finest work.

> Mother used to take me frequently to the market.... The market women were a big, rough, fat, jolly set, who did not know what sickness was, and it might have been well for me if I had stayed among them and grown up like mother. One time in the market-place I saw a totally different set of women. It was about 8 o'clock in the morning, when some people began to shout: "Here come the rich Americans! Now we will sell things!" We saw a large party of travelers coming through the crowd. They looked very queer. Their clothes seemed queer, as they were so different from ours. They wore leather boots instead of

wooden shoes, and they all looked weak and pale. The women were tall and thin, like beanpoles, and their shoulders were stooped and narrow; most of them wore glasses or spectacles, showing that their eyes were weak. The corners of their mouths were all pulled down, and their faces were crossed and crisscrossed with lines and wrinkles, as though they were carrying all the care of the world. Our women all began to laugh and dance and shout at the strangers.... The sight of these people gave me my first idea of America. I heard that the women there never worked, laced themselves too tightly, and were always ill.[278]

The French dressmaker who wrote this passage has the true idea of education and of mind. The mind is an organ for controlling the environment, and it is a safe general principle that the mind which shows high power in the manipulation of a simple situation will show the same quality of efficiency in a more complex one.

The savage, the peasant, the poor man, and woman are not what we call intellectual, because they are not taught to know and manipulate the materials of knowledge. The savage is outside the process from geographical reasons; the peasant is not in the center of interest; the poor man's needs are pressing, and do not permit of interests of a mediate character; and woman does not participate because it is neither necessary nor womanly.

Even the most serious women of the present day stand, in any work they undertake, in precisely the same relation to men that the amateur stands to the professional in games. They may be desperately interested and may work to the limit of endurance at times; but, like the amateur, they got into the game late, and have not had a life-time of practice, or they do not have the advantage of that pace gained only by competing incessantly with players of the very first rank. No one will contend that the amateur in billiards has a nervous organization less fitted to the game than the professional; it is admitted that the difference lies in the constant practice of the professional, the more exacting standards prevailing in the professional ranks, and constant play in "fast company." A group of women would make a sorry spectacle in competition with a set of men who made billiards their life-work. But how sad a spectacle the eminent philosophers of the world would make in the same competition!

Scientific pursuits and the allied intellectual occupations are a game which women have entered late, and their lack of practice is frequently mistaken for lack of natural ability. Writing some years ago of the women in his classes at the University of Zürich, Professor Carl Vogt said:

> At lectures the young women are models of attention and application; perhaps they even make too great effort to carry home in black and white what they have heard. They generally sit in the front seats, because they register early, and, moreover, because they come early, long before the lecture begins. But it is noticeable that they give only a superficial glance at the preparations which the professor passes around. Sometimes they pass them to their neighbor without even looking at them; a longer examination would prevent their taking notes.

> On examination the conduct of the young women is the same as during the lectures. They know better than the young men. To employ a classroom expression, they are enormously crammed. Their memory is good, so that they know perfectly how to give the answer to the question which is put. But generally they stop there. An indirect question makes them lose the thread. As soon as the examiner appeals to individual reason, the examination is over; they do not answer. The examiner seeks to make the sense of the question clearer, and uses a word, perhaps, which is in the manuscript of the student, when, pop! the thing goes as if you had pressed the button of a telephone. If the examination consisted solely in written or oral replies to questions on subjects which have been treated in the lectures or which could be read up on in the manuals, the ladies would always secure brilliant results. But, alas! there are other practical tests in which the candidate finds herself face to face with reality, and that she cannot meet successfully unless she has done practical work in the laboratories, and it is there the shoe pinches.

> The respect in which laboratory work is particularly difficult to women —one would hardly believe it—is that they are often very awkward

and clumsy with their hands. The assistants in the laboratories are unanimous in their complaint; they are pursued with questions about the most trifling things, and one woman gives them more trouble than three men. One would think the delicate fingers of these young women adapted especially to microscopic work, to the manipulation of small slides, to cutting thin sections, to making the most delicate preparations; the truth is quite the contrary. You can tell the table of a woman at a glance: from the fragments of glass, broken instruments, the broken scalpels, the spoiled preparations. There are doubtless exceptions, but they are exceptions.[279]

Zürich was among the first of the European universities opening their doors to women, and it is particularly interesting to see their first efforts in connection with the higher learning. Without a wide experience of life, and without practice in constructive thinking, they naturally fell back on the memory to retain a hold on results in a field with which they were not sufficiently trained to operate in it independently. It is frequently alleged, and is implied in Professor Vogt's report, that women are distinguished by good memories and poor powers of generalization. But this is to mistake the facts. A tenacious memory is characteristic of women and children, and of all persons unskilled in the manipulation of varied experiences in thought. But when the mind is able at any moment to construct a result from the raw materials of experience, the memory loses something of its tenacity and absoluteness. In this sense it may even be said that a good memory for details is a sign of an untrained or imitative mind. As the mind becomes more inventive, the memory is less concerned with the details of knowledge and more with the knowledge of places to find the details when they are needed in any special problem.

The awkwardness in manual manipulation shown by these girls was also surely due to lack of practice. The fastest typewriter in the world is today a woman; the record for roping steers (a feat depending on manual dexterity rather than physical force) is held by a woman; and anyone who will watch girls making change before the pneumatic tubes in the great department stores about Christmas time will experience the same wonder one feels on first seeing a professional gambler shuffling cards.

In short, Professor Vogt's report on women students is just what was to be expected in Germany forty years ago. The American woman, with the enjoyment of greater liberty, has made an approach toward the standards of professional scholarship, and some individuals stand at the very top in their university studies and examinations. The trouble with these cases is that they are either swept away and engulfed by the modern system of marriage, or find themselves excluded in some intangible way from association with men in the fullest sense, and no career open to their talents.

The personal liberty of women is, comparatively speaking, so great in America, suggestion and copies for imitation are spread broadcast so copiously in the schools, newspapers, books, and lectures, and occupations and interests are becoming so varied, that a number of women of natural ability and character are realizing some definite aim in a perfect way. But these are sporadic cases, representing usually some definite interest rather than a full intellectual life, and resembling also in their nature and rarity the elevation of a peasant to a position of eminence in Europe. Nowhere in the world do women as a class lead a perfectly free intellectual life in common with the men of the group, unless it be in restricted and artificial groups like the modern revolutionary party in Russia.

Even in America a number of the great schools are not coeducational, and in those which are so, many of the instructors claim that they do not find it possible to treat with the men and women on precisely the same basis, both because of their own mental attitude toward mixed classes and the inability of the women to receive such treatment. In the case of women also we can say what Mr. Smith says of the Chinese and their system of education, that it is impossible not to marvel at the results they accomplish in view of the system under which they work.

The mind and the personality are largely built up by suggestion from the outside, and if the suggestions are limited and particular, so will be the mind. The world of modern intellectual life is in reality a white man's world. Few women and perhaps no blacks have ever entered this world in the fullest sense. To enter it in the fullest sense would be to be in it at every moment from the time of birth to the time of death, and to absorb it unconsciously and consciously, as the child absorbs language. When something like this happens, we shall be in a position to judge of the mental efficiency of woman and the lower races. At present we seem justified in inferring that the differences in mental expression between the higher and lower races and between men and women are no greater than they should be in view of the existing differences in opportunity.

Indeed, when we take into consideration the superior cunning as well as the superior endurance of women, we may even raise the question whether their capacity for intellectual work is not under equal conditions greater than in men. Cunning is the analogue of constructive thought—an indirect, mediated, and intelligent approach to a problem—and characteristic of the female, in contrast with the more direct and open procedure of the male. Owing to the limited and personal nature of the activities of woman, this trait has expressed itself historically in womankind as intrigue rather than invention, but that it is very deeply based in the instincts is shown by the important rôle it plays in the life of the female in animal life. Endurance is also a factor of prime importance in intellectual performance, for here as in business life "it is doggedness as does it;" and if woman's endurance and natural ingenuity were combined in intellectual pursuits, it might prove that the gray mare is the better horse in this field as well as in peasant life. The most serious objection, also, to the view that woman is fitted to do continuous and hard work, arises from her relation to child-bearing; but this is at bottom trivial. The period of child-bearing is not only not continuous through life, but it is not serious from the standpoint of the time lost. No work is without interruption, and child-birth is an incident in the life of normal woman of no more significance, when viewed in the aggregate and from the standpoint of time, than the interruption of the work of men by their in-and out-of-door games. The important point in all work is not to be uninterrupted, but to begin again.

Whether the characteristic mental life of women and the lower races will prove to be identical with those of the white man or different in quality is a different question, and problematical. It is certain, at any rate, that our civilization is not of the highest type possible. In all our relations there is too much of primitive man's fighting instinct and technique; and it is not impossible that the participation of woman and the lower races will contribute new elements, change the stress of attention, disturb the equilibrium, and force a crisis which will result in the reconstruction of our habits on more sympathetic and equitable principles. Certain it is that no civilization can remain the highest if another civilization adds to the intelligence of its men the intelligence of its women.